Silvia Elizabeth Ferrari

**Detection of anti-ADAMTS13 antibodies in patients with TTP**

Silvia Elizabeth Ferrari

# Detection of anti-ADAMTS13 antibodies in patients with TTP

Characterization of the immune response against ADAMTS13 in patients with thrombotic thrombocytopenic purpura

Südwestdeutscher Verlag für Hochschulschriften

## Impressum / Imprint

Bibliografische Information der Deutschen Nationalbibliothek: Die Deutsche Nationalbibliothek verzeichnet diese Publikation in der Deutschen Nationalbibliografie; detaillierte bibliografische Daten sind im Internet über http://dnb.d-nb.de abrufbar.

Alle in diesem Buch genannten Marken und Produktnamen unterliegen warenzeichen-, marken- oder patentrechtlichem Schutz bzw. sind Warenzeichen oder eingetragene Warenzeichen der jeweiligen Inhaber. Die Wiedergabe von Marken, Produktnamen, Gebrauchsnamen, Handelsnamen, Warenbezeichnungen u.s.w. in diesem Werk berechtigt auch ohne besondere Kennzeichnung nicht zu der Annahme, dass solche Namen im Sinne der Warenzeichen- und Markenschutzgesetzgebung als frei zu betrachten wären und daher von jedermann benutzt werden dürften.

Bibliographic information published by the Deutsche Nationalbibliothek: The Deutsche Nationalbibliothek lists this publication in the Deutsche Nationalbibliografie; detailed bibliographic data are available in the Internet at http://dnb.d-nb.de.

Any brand names and product names mentioned in this book are subject to trademark, brand or patent protection and are trademarks or registered trademarks of their respective holders. The use of brand names, product names, common names, trade names, product descriptions etc. even without a particular marking in this works is in no way to be construed to mean that such names may be regarded as unrestricted in respect of trademark and brand protection legislation and could thus be used by anyone.

Coverbild / Cover image: www.ingimage.com

Verlag / Publisher:
Südwestdeutscher Verlag für Hochschulschriften
ist ein Imprint der / is a trademark of
OmniScriptum GmbH & Co. KG
Heinrich-Böcking-Str. 6-8, 66121 Saarbrücken, Deutschland / Germany
Email: info@svh-verlag.de

Herstellung: siehe letzte Seite /
Printed at: see last page
**ISBN: 978-3-8381-3862-6**

Zugl. / Approved by: Vienna, University of Vienna, Dissertation, 2012

Copyright © 2014 OmniScriptum GmbH & Co. KG
Alle Rechte vorbehalten. / All rights reserved. Saarbrücken 2014

# TABLE OF CONTENTS

TABLE OF CONTENTS ............................................................................... - 1 -
ORIGINAL PUBLICATIONS ....................................................................... - 3 -
LIST OF ABBREVIATIONS .......................................................................... - 5 -
ABSTRACT ..................................................................................................... - 7 -
ZUSAMMENFASSUNG ................................................................................. - 9 -
**1- INTRODUCTION** ................................................................................. - 11 -
  1. Introduction ............................................................................................... - 11 -
    1.1 Overview of Hemostasis ........................................................................ - 11 -
      1.1.1 Primary Hemostasis .......................................................................... - 12 -
      1.1.2 Secondary Hemostasis ...................................................................... - 13 -
  1.2 Von Willebrand Factor ............................................................................ - 16 -
  1.3 ADAMTS13 ............................................................................................ - 18 -
    1.3.1 ADAMTS13 identification and cloning ............................................. - 18 -
    1.3.2 ADAMTS13 biosynthesis, secretion and catabolism ........................ - 18 -
    1.3.3 ADAMTS13 structure and domain organization .............................. - 19 -
    1.3.4 ADAMTS13-VWF interactions and ADAMTS13 activity regulation ..... - 21 -
  1.4 Measurement of ADAMTS13 activity, functional inhibitor and antigen ....... - 24 -
  1.5 Thrombotic thrombocytopenic purpura and the role of ADAMTS13 ............ - 25 -
  1.6 Treatment of thrombotic thrombocytopenic purpura ................................ - 28 -
  1.7 Anti-CD36 antibodies in TTP patients ...................................................... - 29 -

**2- AIM OF THE THESIS** ........................................................................... - 31 -

**3- METHODOLOGY** .................................................................................. - 33 -
  3.1 Patients ................................................................................................... - 33 -
  3.2 Measurement of the ADAMTS13 activity and inhibitor ......................... - 34 -
  3.3 Measurement of ADAMTS13 protein (antigen) levels ........................... - 36 -
  3.4 Detection of anti-ADAMTS13 antibodies ............................................... - 37 -
  3.5 Detection of IgG anti-ADAMTS13 antibodies by a commercial ELISA kit .- 40 -
  3.6 Detection of circulating immune complexes by co-immunoprecipitation and Western blotting ............................................................................................. - 40 -
  3.7 Detection of circulating immune complexes by ELISA .......................... - 41 -
  3.8 Detection of anti-CD36 antibodies by ELISA ......................................... - 43 -

   3.9 Statistical analysis ................................................................................... - 44 -

# 4- RESULTS ............................................................................................. - 45 -
   4.1 Demographic and clinical features of the patients enrolled ......................... - 45 -

   4.2 ADAMTS13 activity, functional ADAMTS13 inhibitor and ADAMTS13 antigen levels in patients with acquired TTP ....................................................... - 46 -

   4.3 Anti-ADAMTS13 antibody profile in patients with acquired TTP ............... - 47 -
      4.3.1 Anti-ADAMTS13 antibody profile in the acute episode ........................ - 47 -
      4.3.2 Correlation between ADAMTS13 antibodies at presentation and ADAMTS13 activity at initial clinical remission ............................................. - 49 -

   4.4 Subclass distribution of IgG anti-ADAMTS13 antibodies ........................... - 49 -
      4.4.1 Subclass distribution of IgG anti-ADAMTS13 antibodies ..................... - 50 -
      4.4.2 Relation between the IgG subclass profile and the total anti-ADAMTS13 IgG antibody titers and ADAMTS13:Ag levels ............................................. - 52 -
      4.4.3 Subclass distribution of anti-ADAMTS13 IgG antibodies and clinical outcome ......................................................................................................... - 54 -

   4.5 Detection of circulating ADAMTS13-anti-ADAMTS13 antibody immune complexes in patients with acquired TTP ......................................................... - 57 -
      4.5.1 Detection of circulating ADAMTS13-anti-ADAMTS13 antibody immune complexes by co-immunoprecipitation .......................................................... - 57 -
      4.5.2 Detection of circulating ADAMTS13-anti-ADAMTS13 antibody immune complexes by ELISA ..................................................................................... - 59 -
      4.5.3 Detection of complement fixing immune complexes by binding to immobilized C1q ........................................................................................... - 61 -

   4.6 Binding of human IgG4 to rabbit anti-ADAMTS13 antibody ...................... - 62 -

   4.7 Detection of anti-ADAMTS13 antibodies and circulating ADAMTS13-immune complexes in a follow-up of a patient with refractory TTP ................................ - 65 -

   4.8 Detection of anti-CD36 antibodies in TTP patients ...................................... - 68 -

# 5- DISCUSSION ....................................................................................... - 70 -

# 6- CONCLUSIONS ................................................................................... - 78 -

# 7- REFERENCES ..................................................................................... - 80 -

# ORIGINAL PUBLICATIONS

Part of this thesis is published in the following manuscripts:

**I.** **Ferrari S**, Scheiflinger F, Rieger M, Mudde G, Wolf M, Coppo P, Girma JP, Azoulay E, Brun-Buisson C, Fakhouri F, Mira JP, Oksenhendler E, Poullin P, Rondeau E, Schleinitz N, Schlemmer B, Teboul JL, Vanhille P, Vernant JP, Meyer D, Veyradier A; French Clinical and Biological Network on Adult Thrombotic Microangiopathies. Prognostic value of anti-ADAMTS 13 antibody features (Ig isotype, titer, and inhibitory effect) in a cohort of 35 adult French patients undergoing a first episode of thrombotic microangiopathy with undetectable ADAMTS 13 activity.
*Blood 2007; 109:2815-22.*

**II.** **Ferrari S**, Mudde GC, Rieger M, Veyradier A, Kremer Hovinga JA, Scheiflinger F. IgG subclass distribution of anti-ADAMTS13 antibodies in patients with acquired thrombotic thrombocytopenic purpura.
*J Thromb Haemost.* 2009; *7:1703-10.*

**III.** **Ferrari S**, Knöbl P, Kolovratova V, Varadi K, Plaimauer B, Turecek P, Rottensteiner H, Scheiflinger F. Inverse correlation of free and immune complexed-sequestred anti-ADAMTS13 antibodies in a patient with acquired TTP.
*J Thromb Haemost.* 2012; 10:*156-8.*

# LIST OF ABBREVIATIONS

| | |
|---|---|
| **ADAMTS13** | A disintegrin-like and metalloprotease with thrombospondin type-1 repeats |
| **ADAMTS13:Ac** | ADAMTS13 activity |
| **ADAMTS13:Ag** | ADAMTS13 antigen |
| **C1q** | Complement component C1q |
| **CD36** | Cluster of differentiation 36 |
| **CUB** | Complement components C1r and C1s, embryonic sea urchin protein (uEGF) and bone morphogenetic protein (Bmp1) domain |
| **ELISA** | Enzyme-linked immunosorbent assay |
| **F** | Coagulation factor |
| **FcγR** | Cell surface Fc gamma receptor |
| **GP** | Glycoprotein |
| **HUS** | Hemolytic uremic syndrome |
| **IC(s)** | Immune complex(es) |
| **Ig** | Immunoglobulin |
| **NHP** | Pooled normal human plasmas |
| **pADAMTS13** | Plasma derived ADAMTS13 |
| **PEX** | Plasma exchange |
| **rADAMTS13** | Recombinant ADAMTS13 |
| **TSP1** | Thrombospondin type 1 motif |
| **TTP** | Thrombotic thrombocytopenic purpura |
| **ULVWF** | Unusually large von Willebrand factor |
| **VWD** | von Willebrand disease |
| **VWF** | von Willebrand factor |

## ABSTRACT

Thrombotic thrombocytopenic purpura (TTP) is a life-threatening disease characterized by microangiopathic hemolytic anemia and thrombocytopenia with renal impairment or neurologic abnormalities due to the deposition of thrombi rich in platelets and von Willebrand factor (VWF) in the microcirculation. ADAMTS13 regulates the size, and therefore the thrombogenic potential, of VWF by cleaving a single peptide bond in VWF. Congenital or acquired ADAMTS13 deficiency is the major risk factor for TTP. Autoantibodies against ADAMTS13 are believed to cause ADAMTS13 deficiency in acquired idiopathic TTP. The main objective of this work was to study the pathophysiologic and prognostic value of anti-ADAMTS13 antibodies in a cohort of 76 patients with acquired TTP. To achieve this goal, enzyme-linked immunosorbent assays were established to detect and quantify IgG1-4, IgA, and IgM anti-ADAMTS13 antibodies as well as circulating ADAMTS13-specific immune complexes (ICs). The surveyed antibody profile revealed the presence of anti-ADAMTS13 antibodies of the IgG, IgA, and IgM class in 92%, 17% and 7% of the patients, respectively. IgG4 (90%) was the most prevalent IgG subclass, followed by IgG1 (52%), IgG2 (50%), and IgG3 (33%). ADAMTS13-specific immune complexes formed by IgG1-4 and IgA were found in 82 and 25% of the patients, respectively. Notably, the complexes contained antibodies of the same Ig (sub)classes as the free antibodies present in most of the samples, being IgG4-ICs the most prevalent (87%) ICs found. Anti-ADAMTS13 IgG antibodies associated with a high inhibitor titer at disease presentation were associated with persistence of undetectable ADAMTS13 activity in clinical remission. TTP patients with high IgG4 and undetectable IgG1 levels were more prone to relapse than patients with low IgG4 and detectable IgG1 levels suggesting that IgG4 could be a useful biomarker for identification of patients at risk of disease recurrence. Circulating ADAMTS13-specific immune complexes may contribute to progression and severity of the disease, because they may continuously deplete ADAMTS13 from circulation inducing organ damage due to tissue deposition. The comprehensive characterization of anti-ADAMTS13 antibodies as well as circulating ADAMTS13-specific ICs is expected to contribute to a better understanding of the mechanisms leading to the autoimmune form of TTP.

## ZUSAMMENFASSUNG

Thrombotische thrombozytopenische Purpura (TTP) ist eine lebensbedrohliche Erkrankung, die durch eine mikroangiopathische Anämie und Thrombozytopenie mit eingeschränkter Nierenfunktion oder neurologischen Auffälligkeiten durch die Ablagerung von Thromben (reich an Thrombozyten und von Willebrand Faktor (VWF)) in der Mikrozirkulation gekennzeichnet ist. ADAMTS13 regelt die Größe und damit das thrombogene Potenzial von VWF durch die Spaltung einer einzigen Peptidbindung in VWF. Angeborener oder erworbener ADAMTS13 Mangel ist der wichtigste Risikofaktor für die TTP. Autoantikörper gegen ADAMTS13 führen vermutlich zum erworbenen ADAMTS13 Mangel in der idiopathischen TTP. Das Hauptziel dieser Arbeit war es, die pathophysiologischen und prognostischen Werte von Anti-ADAMTS13 Antikörpern in einer Kohorte von 76 Patienten mit erworbener TTP zu untersuchen. Deshalb wurden Enzym-gekoppelte Immun-Assays etabliert, die IgG1-4, IgA, IgM-und Anti-ADAMTS13 Antikörper sowie die zirkulierenden ADAMTS13-spezifische Immunkomplexe (ICs) erkennen und quantifizieren können. Das untersuchte Antikörper Profil zeigte die Anwesenheit von anti-ADAMTS13 Antikörper der IgG, IgA, IgM-Klasse in 92%, 17% und 7% der Patienten. IgG4 (90%) war die häufigste IgG Unterklasse gefolgt von IgG1 (52%), IgG2 (50%) und IgG3 (33%). ADAMTS13-spezifische Immunkomplexe, bestehend aus IgG1-4-und IgA, wurden in 82 und 25% der Patienten gefunden. Es ist bemerkenswert, dass diese Immunkomplexe Antikörper der gleichen Ig (sub-) Klassen enthielten wie die in den meisten Proben gefundenen freien Antikörper, wobei IgG4-ICs am häufigsten (87%) ICS vorkamen. Anti-ADAMTS13 IgG-Antikörper, die mit einem hohen Inhibitor-Titer bei Krankheitserscheinung einhergingen, wurden mit nicht nachweisbarer ADAMTS13 Tätigkeit in klinischer Remission assoziiert. TTP Patienten mit hohen IgG4 und nicht nachweisbaren IgG1-Spiegeln waren anfälliger für Krankheitsrückfälle als Patienten mit niedrigen IgG4 und nachweisbaren IgG1-Spiegeln, was darauf hindeutet, dass IgG4 ein nützlicher Biomarker für die Identifizierung von Patienten mit Rezidiv-Risiko sein könnte. Zirkulierende

ADAMTS13-spezifische Immunkomplexe können zur Progression und Schwere der Krankheit beitragen, weil sie kontinuierlich ADAMTS13 aus der Blutzirkulation entfernen, was zu Gewebeablagerungen und nachfolgenden Organschädigungen führt. Die umfassende Charakterisierung von anti-ADAMTS13 Antikörpern sowie zirkulierenden ADAMTS13-spezifischen ICs kann zu einem besseren Verständnis der Mechanismen beitragen, die zu der Autoimmunerkrankungsform der TTP führen.

# 1- INTRODUCTION

## 1. Introduction

ADAMTS13 is the thirteenth member of the ADAMTS (A Disintegrin-like And Metalloprotease with ThromboSpondin type-1 repeats) family of metalloproteases. Its function is to regulate the size of the hemostatic protein von Willebrand factor (VWF)[1]. VWF is released from intracellular storage compartments in the form of multimers containing a portion of very high molecular weight multimers referred to as ultra-large VWF (ULVWF) multimers[2]. These ULVWF multimers bear a high prothrombotic potential, but usually they are proteolyzed by ADAMTS13 immediately after secretion, thereby reducing the size and by consequence the prothrombotic properties of VWF while maintaining its hemostatic function. This function confers to ADAMTS13 an important role in the maintenance of a balanced hemostasis.

## 1.1 Overview of Hemostasis

Hemostasis is a protective physiological mechanism by which the body prevents loss of blood at the site of injury while maintaining normal blood flow elsewhere in the circulation. Hemostasis is a dynamic and complex system, involving cells, coagulation proteins and the vascular wall to keep the blood in a fluid state, but the same players form a barrier when trauma or pathologic conditions cause vessel damage. When the continuity of the vascular endothelium is disrupted, components of the subendothelial layers of the vessel wall are exposed to flowing blood allowing circulating platelets to adhere thereby initiating blood arrest. Activated platelets stimulate the activation of plasma coagulation factors leading to the generation of fibrin that stabilizes the platelet plug. Fibrin also provides a matrix for cell migration and wound healing. In the latter case, the platelet aggregate and fibrin clot are dissolved and removed by the fibrinolytic system which completes the process of hemostasis[3].

Hemostasis is a tightly regulated process. In the absence of injury, regulatory mechanisms ensure the maintenance of blood fluidity. After tissue damage the system is immediately activated. As a consequence a thrombus is generated that remains localized to the site of injury and is proportional to the size of injury[4]. A balance between procoagulant and anticoagulant pathways is critical to achieve a regulated hemostasis[4]. Disturbances of the natural balance due to genetic or acquired factors may result in either bleeding (not enough clotting) or thrombosis (too much clotting).

Hemostasis can be divided into primary and secondary hemostasis. Primary hemostasis is mediated by platelets which aggregate to form a hemostatic plug at the site of injury. Secondary hemostasis is the generation of insoluble fibrin by the coagulation cascade. Both processes occur simultaneously and are mechanistically intertwined[4;5].

## 1.1.1 Primary Hemostasis

The intact vascular endothelium is a non-adhesive surface with which platelets are not interacting under normal blood flow. However, when the endothelium is disrupted by mechanical damage (traumatic wounds) or pathogenic stimuli (e.g. chronic vascular diseases), extracellular matrix (ECM) components become exposed to circulating blood triggering events of primary hemostasis. Platelet adhesion is the first response to vascular injury and is an important host defense mechanism to avoid bleeding. Platelet adhesion requires the synergistic and coordinated function of different plasma proteins and receptors on platelets together with ECM components[6].

The initial platelet tethering to the vessel wall is mediated by the interaction between two platelet surface receptors (glycoprotein (GP) VI and integrin $\alpha 2\beta 1$) and subendothelial collagen. Subendothelial VWF also mediates platelet adhesion by binding to the platelet receptors GPIb$\alpha$ (platelet membrane GPIb-IX-V complex)[7] and integrin $\alpha IIb\beta 3$[8]. Soluble plasma VWF can also be immobilized to ECM components via direct binding to sudendothelial collagen or self-association with other VWF multimers, thus acting as a bridge between tissue and platelets[6;9].

After platelets are firmly adhered to ECM components, they can translocate on the injured vessel wall and on the surface of the developing thrombus. This step is critical for the regulation of the rate and extent of thrombus growth. Platelet translocation also generates signals that induce platelet morphological changes like rearrangement of the membrane with exposure of negatively charged phospholipids and development of tethers/pseudopodia that increase the platelet potential to establish multivalent adhesive interactions[10;11]. The exposition of negatively charged phospholipids (mainly phosphatidylserine) on the outer membrane layer of platelets is particularly critical for platelet procoagulant activity. Platelet activation and granule content release are responsible for activation of additional platelets[10]. Platelet activation also stimulates integrin $\alpha IIb\beta 3$ activation, enhancing its affinity for adhesive proteins such as soluble fibrinogen, VWF, fibronectin and thrombospondin[12]. Fibrinogen physically bridges adjacent activated platelets promoting cell arrest and stable platelet aggregation. Platelet aggregation mediated by binding of soluble fibrinogen to platelet integrin αIIbβ3 is the dominant mechanism supporting platelet aggregation under low wall shear rate conditions (0 to 1000 $s^{-1}$). With increasing wall shear rates (1000 to 10 000 $s^{-1}$), the initiation of aggregation becomes more dependent on VWF and fibrinogen only supports the stabilization of the formed aggregates[11]. Nevertheless, fibrinogen and VWF have a synergistic role supporting platelet aggregation and both are required to ensure a stable primary plug. Primary hemostasis is coordinated with the activation of the coagulation system (secondary hemostasis) which will generate thrombin and deposition of an insoluble fibrin net stabilizing and anchoring the primary thrombus to the vessel wall.

## 1.1.2 Secondary Hemostasis

The original waterfall/cascade model of coagulation depicted as a Y-shaped scheme was described in 1964 independently by Davie and Ratnoff[13] and Macfarlane[14]. This model describes a complex series of sequential enzymatic reactions in which several inactive plasma coagulation zymogens are converted to active serine proteases along either an extrinsic or an intrinsic pathway that converge at a common pathway that ends with the generation of thrombin and a fibrin clot (Fig.1).

The activation of the extrinsic pathway is triggered by the exposition of tissue factor (TF) to flowing blood, which occurs after vascular damage or activation of the endothelium. Tissue factor is a transmembrane protein constitutively expressed on cells that are not in contact with blood. TF binds to activated plasma factor (F) VII (FVIIa, with the lower case "a" indicating active clotting factor), about ~1% of which circulates as active enzyme. Circulating FVIIa displays a weak catalytic activity that is enhanced only when bound to TF, calcium ions and membrane surfaces to form the catalytic TF/FVIIa tenase complex. TF/FVIIa complex activates the zymogens FIX (belonging to the intrinsic pathway) and FX to their active forms (IXa and Xa, respectively)[15]. At this initial stage, trace amounts of thrombin are generated by the minute quantities of FXa produced. The small amount of thrombin generated is not sufficient to induce clot formation but will partially activate platelets and the cofactors FV and FVIII to their active forms allowing the propagation and amplification of the coagulation to generate a fibrin clot[16] (Fig.1).

Initiation of the intrinsic pathway is triggered by the autoactivation of plasma coagulation factor XII upon contact with negatively charged biological or artificial surfaces (e.g. platelet membrane, collagen, glass) by a process called "contact activation". In the presence of high-molecular-weight kininogen (HMWK), a platelet-derived cofactor, small amounts of FXIIa can convert prekallikrein into active kallikrein which reciprocally activates more FXII thereby amplifying the activation signal. Factor XIIa, in the presence of HMWK, proteolytically cleaves FXI to FXIa which in turn activates FIX to FIXa[17;18].

Factor IXa assembles with activated FVIII (FVIIIa) and calcium ions into a complex on negatively charged platelet membranes. This so called tenase complex catalyzes the activation of FX to FXa (Fig.1).

The extrinsic and intrinsic pathways converge at the step of FX activation. In the common pathway, FXa forms a complex with FVa, calcium ions and phospholipid membranes (prothrombinase complex) which activates prothrombin to thrombin (FIIa). Thrombin converts fibrinogen to fibrin monomers that spontaneously polymerize in a soft and friable clot (Fig.1). Furthermore, thrombin activates FXIII to FXIIIa which catalyzes the formation of covalent cross-links between fibrin polymers to form a fibrin mesh thus enhancing clot stability and resistance[19].

The waterfall/cascade model of coagulation supports the in vitro evaluation of coagulation function but may not explain coagulation in vivo. The catalytic reactions of blood coagulation are localized on phospholipid surfaces mainly provided by platelets, but cells also play a key role in controlling and directing the coagulation event to avoid its spreading throughout the vascular system. A modified cell-based model of coagulation has been proposed which describes the interaction of clotting factors with specific cell surfaces in an overlapping manner and not only in a sequential cascade of reactions[20;21].

In this cell-based model, coagulation occurs in three overlapping phases: initiation, amplification and propagation[20;21]. The initiation of coagulation is driven in vivo by the extrinsic or TF-dependent pathway that includes the FVIIa/TF and the FXa/FVa complexes and operates exclusively on TF-bearing cells. During this phase, the FVIIa/TF complex activates FIX and FX. FIXa is able to migrate to other cellular surfaces whereas FXa remains on TF-bearing cells, where it activates FV to form the FXa/FVa or prothrombinase complex, which in turn produces small amounts of thrombin. These small quantities of thrombin suffice to activate platelets, FV, FVIII and FXI, thereby initiating the amplification phase. This phase occurs mainly on platelets and ends with the binding of FVa and FVIIIa to the surface of activated platelets. In the propagation phase, the tenase complex (FVIIIa/FIXa) bound to platelet membranes activates FX, which will form the prothrombinase complex (FXa/FVa) on the platelet surface. This complex generates a large amount of thrombin, which finally converts fibrinogen to fibrin and activates FXIII leading to a stabilization of the forming clot[20;21].

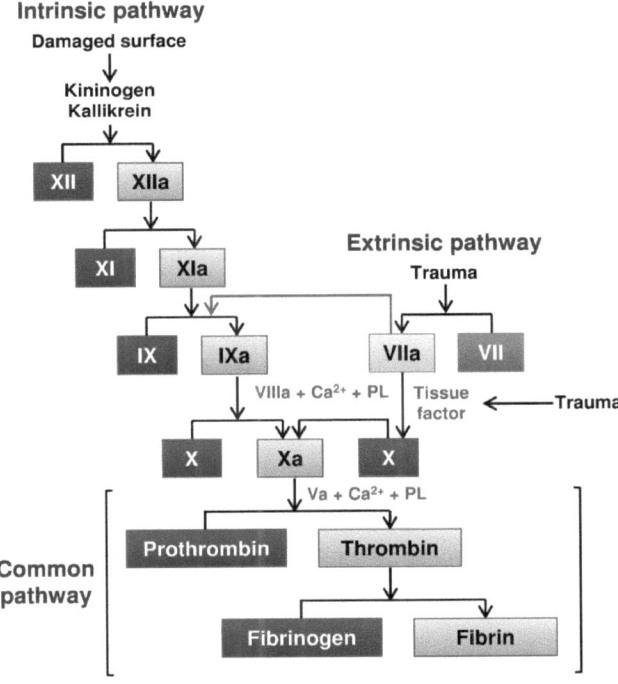

**Figure 1. Schematic representation of the coagulation cascade.**

The intrinsic and extrinsic pathways are depicted. Plasma coagulation zymogens are indicated by roman numbers and activated factors by a lower case "a". Non-enzymatic cofactors are indicated in green. The red line indicates a reaction that does not belong to the standard waterfall cascade described in 1964.

On the other hand, contact activation does not play any physiological role in that process. The intrinsic pathway is only operating on platelet surfaces and is driven by FXIa and the tenase (FVIIIa/FIXa) and prothrombinase (FXa/FVa) complexes.

According to this model, both pathways are required to achieve hemostasis because they work on different cell surfaces having different functional roles.

## 1.2 Von Willebrand Factor

The von Willebrand factor is a large plasma multimeric glycoprotein that exerts two important biological functions. In primary hemostasis, VWF supports platelet adhesion and aggregation[6]. The second relevant function of VWF relates to its role in secondary hemostasis, as it serves as a carrier protein for the procoagulant plasma factor VIII. VWF forms a complex with FVIII via non-covalent interactions increasing the plasma half-life of FVIII and conferring protection from proteolytic degradation[22].

VWF is synthesized exclusively in megakaryocytes[23] and endothelial cells[24]. The VWF precursor protein (denoted as pre-pro-VWF) consists of a monomeric polypeptide of 2813 amino acids with a molecular weight of about 350 kDa. The structure of pre-pro-VWF is based on a 22 amino acid signal peptide, a pro-peptide comprising 741 residues and a mature subunit of 2050 amino acids. The pro-VWF is composed of four types of repeated domains (A to D) displaying considerable internal homology and linked in the order: NH2-D1-D2-D'-D3-A1-A2-A3-D4-B1-B2-B3-C1-C2-CK-COOH. Each domain contains different physiological binding functions. Domains D1 and D2 correspond to the VWF propeptide whereas mature VWF is composed of domains D' to CK[25;26].

Pro-VWF is extensively post-translationally modified to produce multimeric VWF. In the endoplasmic reticulum, pro-VWF monomers dimerize in a 'tail-to-tail' manner through disulfide bonds within the C-terminal domains. In the Golgi apparatus, pro-VWF dimers polymerize via additional N-terminal 'head-to-head' disulfide bonds yielding high molecular weight multimeric VWF species, the sizes of which can reach molecular weights up to 20.000 kDa or even higher. Multimer assembly is promoted by the VWF-propeptide which is proteolytically cleaved from the VWF subunits inside the *trans*-Golgi. The VWF-propeptide is also required to direct and package VWF multimers into specialized storage organelles, the so-called Weibel-Palade bodies of endothelial cells and the α-granules of megakaryocytes and platelets.

In endothelial cells, VWF multimers are secreted immediately after synthesis from both cellular sides (apical and basal) via a constitutive pathway or stored in the Weibel-Palade bodies and released after induction with secretagogues via a regulated pathway[25] or, probably, by an unstimulated basal pathway[27]. In contrast, VWF stored in megakaryocytes and platelets is secreted only upon activation via the regulated pathway[28].

VWF is released from the stored compartments in the form of multimers containing a portion of very high molecular weight multimers referred to as ultra-large VWF (ULVWF) multimers[2]. These highest molecular weight VWF species are the hemostatically most active forms with a propensity to promote spontaneous platelet adhesion and aggregation under high shear. As this aggregation can occur even in the absence of endothelial damage ULVW multimers bear a significant prothrombotic potential[29].

VWF multimer size is regulated by ADAMTS13 (A Disintegrin-like And Metalloprotease with ThromboSpondin type-1 repeats), a metalloprotease that specifically cleaves the peptide bond between the amino acids Tyr1605 and Met1606 within the central A2 domain of VWF[30;31]. This conversion of the ULVWF multimers to smaller and less active forms is thought to predominantly occur immediately after secretion of VWF.

The first association between the presence of circulating ULVWF multimers and thrombosis was made in 1982[32] in a description of patients suffering of chronic relapsing thrombotic thrombocytopenic purpura (TTP), a life-threatening thrombotic microangiopathy characterized by thrombocytopenia, microangiopathic hemolytic anemia and renal impairment or neurological abnormalities. The ULVWF multimers were present in the plasma only during the remission phase of the disease, disappearing after fresh plasma replacement or during the acute phase. This led to the speculation that ULVWF multimers are responsible for the widespread thrombus formation observed in the microvasculature of the patients and that a plasma deficiency of a VWF depolymerase (today known as ADAMTS13) could be the cause of the accumulation of ULVWF multimers.

On the other hand, deficiency of VWF can cause a bleeding disorder called von Willebrand disease (VWD). VWD is the most common autosomally inherited bleeding disorder due to quantitative (type 1 and 3) or qualitative (type 2) deficiencies of VWF[33]. In type 1 VWD, VWF levels are partially reduced, whereas in type 3 VWD are undetectable. Type 2 VWD is characterized by qualitative defects in VWF that lead to impaired protein function and can be divided into four different subclasses (2A, 2B, 2M and 2N) based on specific functional and structural defects. Patients with type 2A VWD have decreased VWF-dependent platelet adhesion due to a selective deficiency of high-molecular-weight VWF multimers. A VWF with increased affinity for platelet GPIb characterize type 2B VWD. Patients with type 2M VWD have decreased VWF-dependent platelet adhesion without a selective deficiency of high-molecular-weight VWF multimers. Finally, a VWF with markedly decreased binding affinity for FVIII characterize type 2N VWD[33].

## 1.3 ADAMTS13
### 1.3.1 ADAMTS13 identification and cloning

Two independent groups partially purified a ~200 kDa plasma protease in 1996 that was capable of cleaving VWF at a single specific site producing the same cleavage fragments of 140 and 176 kDa as observed in normal human plasma[30;31]. The newly identified protease cleaved VWF only after exposure to mild denaturation with chaotropic agents such as urea[30] and guanidine-HCl[31] or to high fluid shear stress[31]. The VWF-cleaving protease (VWFCP) was found to be activated by divalent cation ions and low ionic strength, strongly inhibited by chelating agents and insensitive to serine and cysteine proteinase inhibitors. Later on, deficiency of the VWFCP was found in patients suffering from chronic relapsing TTP[34] and it was shown that in some cases, an isolated IgG from plasma of TTP patients inhibited the proteolytic activity of the VWFCP, suggesting that a constitutional or acquired deficiency of the VWFCP has led to development of TTP[35;36].

In 2001, the VWFCP was isolated, cloned and identified as a new member of the ADAMTS (A Disintegrin-like And Metalloprotease with ThromboSpondin type-1 repeats) metalloprotease family, designed ADAMTS13[37-42].

The human *ADAMTS13* gene contains 29 exons encompassing approximately 37kb on human chromosome 9q34. The 4.7 kb transcript encoded by the *ADAMTS13* gene is predominantly expressed in the liver and a short 2.4 kb transcript was also found in placenta and skeletal muscles[39-41].

### 1.3.2 ADAMTS13 biosynthesis, secretion and catabolism

ADAMTS13 is synthesized in the hepatic stellate cells of the liver[43;44], platelets[45], endothelial cells[46] and podocytes and renal tubular epithelial cells from the kidney[47;48]. In contrast to other ADAMTS proteases, ADAMTS13 is secreted into the circulation as an active enzyme[49] with a plasma half-life of approximately 2-3 days[50]. The estimated normal plasma concentration of ADAMTS13 is ~1 μg/ml (5 nM)[37;51]. A small percentage (~3%) of ADAMTS13 circulates bound to native VWF without exerting substrate proteolysis[52].

Full length ADAMTS13 is the major plasma circulating species, however, truncated forms have also been identified[37;53]. Mature ADAMTS13 is highly posttranslationally modified with glycosylation accounting for ~20% of its molecular weight. N-glycosylation[54] and O-fucosylation of the TSP1 repeats[55] seem to be critical for ADAMTS13 secretion based on studies in cell culture with recombinantly expressed ADAMTS13. Moreover, N-glycosylation seems to be important for promoting a correct protein folding rendering ADAMTS13 proteolytically more active. N-glycans are however not required for protease activity once ADAMTS13 is correctly folded and secreted[54]. Using purified plasma-derived ADAMTS13 (pADAMTS13), Hiura *et al*[56] showed that ADAMTS13 contains α2-6 and α2-3-linked sialic acid residues at the non-reducing terminus and β-galactose residues on the N- and O-linked sugar chains penultimate to sialic acid.

The mechanism by which ADAMTS13 is cleared or metabolized in vivo is unknown. Recent findings indicate that all sugar chains of pADAMTS13 are capped by sialic acids with no exposure of galactose residues. This could suggest that the hepatic asialoglycoprotein receptor is involved in ADAMTS13 clearance[56]. It has been reported that thrombin, plasmin and factor Xa can inactivate ADAMTS13 in vitro[57]. Leucocyte elastase also cleaves pADAMTS13 but at sites different from those of thrombin and plasmin[56]. These results suggest that ADAMTS13 activity might be locally regulated by coagulation proteinases.

### 1.3.3 ADAMTS13 structure and domain organization

ADAMTS13 is a protein with a multidomain structure (Fig. 2). The primary ADAMTS13 sequence consists of a polypeptide with 1427 amino acid residues sharing common domains with other members of the ADAMTS family. At its N-terminus, ADAMTS13 harbors a 33 amino acid signal peptide and a short propeptide (residues 34-74). The mature sequence consists of a reprolysin-like metalloprotease domain (residues 75-289), a disintegrin-like domain (residues 290-385), a central thrombospondin type 1 (TSP1-1) motif (residues 386-439), a cysteine-rich domain (residues 440-555), a spacer domain (residues 556-685) followed by a unique combination of seven additional TSP1 repeats (TSP1 2-8; residues 686-1131) and two CUB domains (residues 1192-1408) which were first identified in complement components C1r and C1s, embryonic sea urchin protein (uEGF) and bone morphogenetic protein (Bmp1).

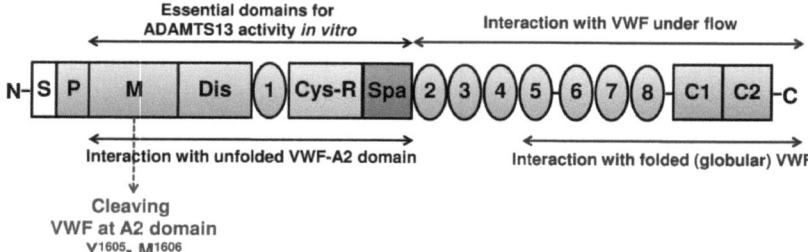

**Figure 2. Schematic diagram of the ADAMTS13 domain structure and proposed VWF interaction sites.**
The domains are indicated from the N-terminus as follows: signal peptide (S), propeptide (P), metalloprotease domain (M), disintegrin-like domain (Dis), the first thrombospondin type 1 motif (TSP1-1), cysteine-rich domain (Cys-R), spacer domain (Spa), the second to eighth TSP1 repeats (2-8) and two CUB domains (C1 and C2). In the metalloprotease domain resides the active site responsible for VWF cleavage. The contributions of the different domains to the binding of ADAMTS13 to folded and unfolded VWF are also depicted.

The crystal structure of full-length ADAMTS13 has not yet been resolved, but that of a fragment comprising the disintegrin-like, TSP1-1, cysteine-rich and spacer domains, all of which are relevant for ADAMTS13 activity, was published recently[58]. In some of these domains peripheral loops were identified that are not conserved among the different members of the ADAMTS family. Identification of these non-conserved domains not only helped to better understand the various interactions between ADAMTS13 and VWF but also suggested that these may confer specific functions to each ADAMTS member[58].

The ADAMTS13 propeptide lacks the cysteine-switch motif present in all other ADAMTS members[40]. Since this motif confers enzyme latency its absence might be responsible for the secretion of ADAMTS13 as an active enzyme[49]. The propeptide is also not required for protein folding and secretion, and its cleavage is not critical for proteolytic activity[49].

The metalloprotease or catalytic domain of ADAMTS13 is responsible for the specific cleavage of VWF and contains the conserved active site motif $^{224}\underline{\text{H}}E XX\underline{\text{H}}XXGXX\underline{\text{HD}}^{235}$ ("X" represent any amino acid). The active site pocket has three histidine residues coordinating a $Zn^{2+}$ ion and a glutamic acid coordinating a water molecule being essential for ADAMTS13 catalytic activity[59]. In addition, the active site has also a conserved Met[249] in a proposed "Met turn" [59] and a predicted high-affinity $Ca^{2+}$-binding site adjacent to the active site cleft[60].

The Cys-rich domain of ADAMTS13 has an RGD sequence that is usually used for recognition of integrins on cellular membranes and could therefore act as a potential anchor to cell surfaces, but this possibility has not yet been investigated.

The thrombospondin-like repeats are homologous to the type I repeats of thrombospondin 1 and 2. The TSPs contain six potential CD36 binding motifs and preliminary in vitro studies showed that ADAMTS13 binds to CD36 via its TSPs without affecting its proteolytic activity suggesting that TSPs may localize ADAMTS13 to the cell surface of endothelial cells[61].

The CUB domains are unique for ADAMTS13[40] and seem to be involved in apical sorting of ADAMTS13 in human endothelial cells and Madin-Darby canine kidney fibroblasts (a well-established cell line for polarized cell) by interacting with membrane lipid rafts[62]. Moreover, CUB domains seem to be critical for recognition and cleavage of VWF under flow conditions[63;64]. Four of five cysteine residues in the CUB-1 domain seem to have a critical role in ADAMTS13 secretion and stability[65].

## 1.3.4 ADAMTS13-VWF interactions and ADAMTS13 activity regulation

VWF is the only known substrate of ADAMTS13 thus conferring to ADAMTS13 a highly selective role. ADAMTS13 cleaves VWF at a single site between amino acids Tyr1605 and Met1606 in the central part of the A2 domain. VWF circulates in a native globular-shaped conformation where the ADAMTS13 cleavage site inside the A2 domain is buried, rendering it inaccessible for ADAMTS13[66]. Partial or complete VWF A2 domain unfolding is required for ADAMTS13 to cleave VWF. In vitro, unfolding is obtained by the use of mild denaturing agents such as urea or guanidine-HCl. In vivo, unfolding is induced by flow under high shear stress as found in small arteries and capillaries. Under flow conditions, newly released ULVWF from Weibel-Palade bodies or endothelial cells remains anchored to the cellular surface via P-selectin[67] or $\alpha_V\beta_3$ integrin[68] in the form of string-like structures that are rapidly cleaved by ADAMTS13. Recent in vitro findings suggest that this type of VWF hardly requires shear stress[69;70]. Cleavage of endothelial cell-anchored ULVWF multimers by ADAMTS13 appears to be the prevalent mechanism in vivo[71;72], but a portion of VWF is likely to be also cleaved in the microcirculation.

ADAMTS13 can also act as disulfide bond reductase of VWF multimers[73]. This novel activity of ADAMTS13 selectively targets inter-molecular disulfide bonds formed between VWF multimers under conditions of high fluid shear stress without affecting bonds that maintain the VWF multimeric structure. This reductase activity seems to be independent of the proteolytic activity of ADAMTS13 and might prevent covalent lateral VWF multimer association, a mechanism that in the absence of ADAMTS13 may lead to an enhanced binding to platelets.

Many cofactors can positively or negatively modulate ADAMTS13 proteolytic activity against VWF by binding to the enzyme itself or to VWF. Cations like $Zn^{2+}$ and $Ca^{2+}$ individually and cooperatively enhance ADAMTS13 proteolytic activity in static assays[74]. Under high shear stress conditions, both platelets[75] and coagulation FVIII[76] independently, or synergistically when added together[77], accelerate and enhance VWF cleavage by ADAMTS13 in vitro. On the other hand, anions ($ClO_4^-$ > $Cl^-$ > $F^-$) may negatively modulate ADAMTS13 activity by binding to VWF under both static and flow conditions[78;79].

During systemic inflammation, several reactive oxygen species are generated which cause oxidative stress that may oxidize the methionine residue at the VWF peptide bond cleavage site ($Met^{1606}$) rendering VWF more resistant to ADAMTS13 proteolysis[80;81]. This effect may generate a prothrombotic state with accumulation of ULVWF multimers in circulation without altering their interaction with platelets.

Multiple interactions between ADAMTS13 and the unfolded VWF A2 domain are required for an efficient and specific proteolysis. The unfolded VWF A2 domain exposes different exosite-binding regions (adjacent and also distant to the cleavage site) that are recognized by counterpart exosites localized within different ADAMTS13 domains favoring a precise positioning of the ADAMTS13 active site next to the target VWF peptide bond.

The contribution of the different domains to the proteolytic activity of ADAMTS13 has been investigated using C-terminally truncated ADAMTS13 fragments. The metalloprotease domain alone showed no proteolytic activity against VWF, and truncations upstream of the spacer domain cleaved full-length VWF with only very low efficacy under static[82-84] and also under flow conditions[85]. Addition of the spacer region restored activity to levels similar to those of full-length ADAMTS13[82-85], highlighting the functional importance of the spacer domain for ADAMTS13 activity. Addition of domains C-terminal to the spacer domain do not further increase the proteolytic activity of ADAMTS13 against VWF[82;83].

The minimal functional VWF substrate identified for ADAMTS13 comprises 73 amino acid residues (Asp1596 to Arg1668) of the C-terminal region of the A2 domain (abbreviated VWF73)[86].

Upon unfolding of the VWF A2 domain the ADAMTS13 spacer domain is docking to residues localized at the C-terminal end of the VWF A2 domain. Amino acids Arg658, Arg660, Tyr661 and Tyr665 within the spacer domain interact with residues between Glu1660 and Arg1668 in the VWF A2 domain[58;84;87-89]. This step seems to be critical for recognition and subsequent cleavage of VWF. Docking of the spacer domain is followed by the binding of residues within the ADAMTS13 disintegrin-like domain close to the VWF cleavage site, thus positioning the VWF cleavage site next to the ADAMTS13 active site[90]. Before proteolysis of VWF can finally occur, subsites within the metalloprotease domain of ADAMTS13 need to interact with VWF residues adjacent to the cleavage site to ensure a highly specific cleavage of the VWF peptide bond[83;87;91]. Finally, stable interactions between the metalloprotease and the disintegrin-like domain appear to be essential for ADAMTS13 activity[58]. The combined observations suggest that efficient substrate recognition, binding and cleavage require multiple N-terminal domains of ADAMTS13.

A productive proteolysis additionally depends on interactions of VWF with the C-terminal domains of ADAMTS13. The first CUB domain (CUB-1) or peptides derived thereof were shown to partially inhibit the docking and cleavage of VWF by ADAMTS13 under static and flow conditions[63]. Moreover, removal of the distal TSP1 2-8 and CUB domains also reduced the binding and cleavage of VWF under flow conditions, suggesting a critical role of these domains in VWF recognition[64;92]. Studies conducted with congenic mice expressing a shorter version of ADAMTS13 that lacks the TSP1 7-8 and CUB domains have demonstrated that these mice were more prone to thrombosis than mice carrying the wild type ADAMTS13 gene, suggesting an impaired capacity of the C-terminally truncated ADAMTS13 to regulate thrombus formation[93]. In vivo studies using ADAMTS13 knockout mice showed that injection of murine (m) ADAMTS13 variants lacking the two CUB domains abolished proteolysis of platelet-decorated VWF strings[94]. Additional injection of truncated mADAMTS13 variants lacking the TSP1 2-8 repeats restored proteolysis. These studies stressed the relevant role of the TSP repeats and CUB domains for ADAMTS13 binding and cleavage of VWF in vivo[94].

## 1.4 Measurement of ADAMTS13 activity, functional inhibitor and antigen

The normal plasma ADAMTS13 activity in healthy individuals ranges from 50-150%. The most widely used laboratory assays to measure ADAMTS13 activity in plasma employ multimeric VWF (purified plasma-derived or recombinant) as substrate and measure directly (by electrophoresis) or indirectly (platelet aggregation, enzyme-linked immunosorbent assay (ELISA)) the degraded VWF products generated after incubation with ADAMTS13[30;31;95-97]. Overall, these assays have moderate sensitivity but they are cumbersome, time-consuming, call for expert laboratory handling and importantly, they measure ADAMTS13 activity under static and non-physiological conditions requiring long incubation times and denaturing conditions (urea or guanidine hydrochloride) to unfold VWF and to mimic the role of the physiological blood shear stress.

Assays using as substrate recombinant VWF domains or short VWF A2 domain-derived peptides have also been developed[98;99]. Most of these assays use the 73 amino acid sequence of VWF (VWF73) shown to be the minimal functional ADAMTS13 substrate[86]. The main advantage of this type of assays is that it does not require denaturing conditions. Currently, the most widely used assay is a fluorescence resonance energy transfer (FRET)-based assay employing a fluorogenic VWF73 as substrate (FRETS-VWF73)[100]. The FRETS-VWF73 assay, although using a non-physiological VWF substrate, showed good agreement with ADAMTS13 activity assays employing full-length VWF[101-103]. It shows high reproducibility and accuracy and requires short incubation times (~1 h).

The measurement of ADAMTS13 functional inhibitor is based on the principle of the Bethesda method originally described for anti-factor VIII antibodies[104]. Heat-inactivated patient and pooled normal plasmas are mixed in a 1:1 proportion and incubated for 2 hours at 37°C. After incubation, the residual ADAMTS13 activity in the mixture is assayed by any of the conventional assays described above. A patient is considered to have an ADAMTS13 functional inhibitor if the residual ADAMTS13 activity in the mixture is less than 75% of a control mixture made with pooled normal plasma and buffer.

A method for measuring ADAMTS13 activity in vitro under flow conditions uses ULVWF multimers secreted by histamine-stimulated endothelial cells as VWF source[71]. This assay seems to be reliable in discriminating ADAMTS13 activity only at levels higher than 20%[105]. Although this assay mimics the in vivo situation more closely as it takes into consideration the endothelial cells and the fluid shear stress, expert laboratory handling is required making it unsuitable for routine testing.

Recently, a vortex-based assay to quantify ADAMTS13 activity and inhibitors has been proposed[106]. According to the authors, the vortex rotation generates a shear stress similar to that found in arteries and appears to be sufficient to unfold and cleave VWF thus mimicking more closely the in vivo situation.

ELISA-based assays to quantify ADAMTS13 antigen levels have been developed using polyclonal[51] or monoclonal[107;108] anti-ADAMTS13 antibodies. When comparing the performance of two of these assays in a multicenter study[109], a good reproducibility and linearity could be demonstrated, with a limit of detection of 10% and 5%, using monoclonal[107] and polyclonal[51] antibodies, respectively.

## 1.5 Thrombotic thrombocytopenic purpura and the role of ADAMTS13

Thrombotic microangiopathies (TMA) are a group of syndromes that share the common features of thrombocytopenia and microangiopathic hemolytic anemia with erythrocyte fragmentation (schistocytes) and increased serum levels of the intracellular enzyme lactate dehydrogenase (LDH)[110]. The classical diseases associated with TMA are thrombotic thrombocytopenic purpura (TTP) and hemolytic uremic syndrome (HUS) although TMA is also observed in a wide range of other diseases such as systemic lupus erythematosus (SLE), malignancy, disseminating intravascular coagulopathy, pre-eclampsia, and endothelial damage due to drug toxicity[111;112].

The HUS is characterized by a triad of renal failure, thrombocytopenia and non-immune hemolytic anemia with schistocytes. The common form of HUS, called typical HUS, is triggered by infection with shiga toxin-producing bacteria and is associated with a favorable outcome. The atypical HUS is a less common form (about 10% of the cases) and is associated with poor prognosis. In 50% of the cases, the atypical HUS is associated with genetic deficiency of the complement regulator protein factors H, I, and B or of membrane cofactor proteins. In the remaining cases, the etiology is unknown[111;112].

TTP is a rare but life-threatening TMA first described by Moschcowitz in 1924[113]. The clinical presentation of TTP is characterized by a pentad of signs and symptoms including fever, thrombocytopenia, microangiopathic hemolytic anemia with red cell fragmentation and renal failure and/or fluctuating neurological abnormalities[114]. A deficiency in plasma ADAMTS13 is the currently accepted pathophysiological mechanism of TTP (Fig. 3). ADAMTS13 deficiency leads to the accumulation of ULVWF multimers under the high shear stress of the microcirculation with subsequent spontaneous platelet adhesion and aggregation and occlusive microvascular thrombosis. The presence of widespread hyaline VWF- and platelet-rich thrombi in the microcirculation causing multiple organ ischemia are the main histopathological features found in TTP patients[114] (Fig. 3).

Even if the pentad of clinical symptoms was originally required as diagnostic criterion for TTP, in the current practice, only the presence of a non-immune microangiopathic hemolytic anemia and thrombocytopenia without any alternative etiology are often sufficient criteria to suggest TTP and prompt initiation of treatment to reduce fatal outcomes[114;115]. Since the introduction of plasma exchange (PEX) with plasma replacement in 1991[116] as first choice therapy, the mortality rate of TTP has been reduced from 90% to 10-20%[117]. The mortality is mainly due to treatment refractoriness. Relapse occurs in 30-50% of the patients who survive an initial episode of TTP, being more often during the first year after the onset[118].

TTP has an estimated annual incidence in the adult population of 4-11 cases per million[119;120]. TTP occurs more frequently in adults than in children and it affects both sexes with an increased incidence for women and black race[119].

Congenital and acquired TTP are the two clinically recognized forms of TTP. Distinction at clinical presentation between these two forms is important because of differences in treatment modalities. Congenital TTP, also known as Upshaw-Schulman Syndrome, is caused by a genetic deficiency of ADAMTS13[41;121], whereas autoantibody-mediated ADAMTS13 deficiency is considered to be the principal cause of acquired idiopathic TTP[35;36] and is often associated with a severe ADAMTS13 deficiency (<10%)[122;123].

A secondary, non-idiopathic acquired form of TTP occurs in association with pregnancy, certain drugs (e.g. ticlopidine, clopidogrel, quinine, chemotherapeutic and immunosuppressive agents), autoimmune disorders, infections, cancer and after hematopoietic stem cell transplantation[115;124]. These cases are rarely associated with severe ADAMTS13 deficiency except for those associated with pregnancy, autoimmune diseases or ticlopidine/clopidogrel treatment[125].

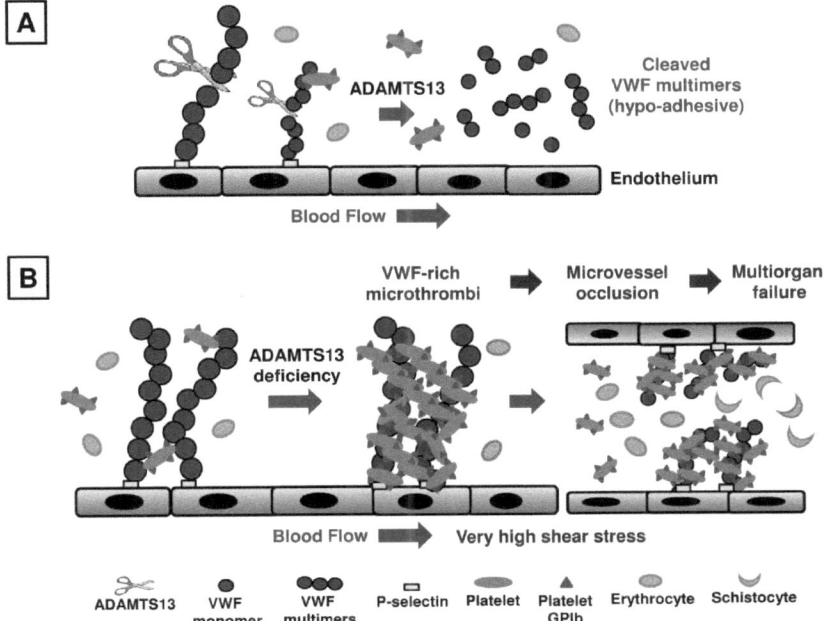

**Figure 3. Role of ADAMTS13 in hemostasis**

(A) Physiological role of ADAMTS13 in hemostasis. VWF multimers bind to endothelial cells (P-selectin) or to exposed extracellular matrix components. Platelets adhere to VWF through glycoprotein GPIb forming a platelet-rich thrombus the growth of which is limited by the proteolytic activity of ADAMTS13. (B) Pathogenesis of thrombotic thrombocytopenic purpura (TTP) caused by ADAMTS13 deficiency. In the absence of ADAMTS13, VWF-dependent platelet accumulation proceeds and eventually causes microvessel occlusion. This will lead to thrombosis and multiorgan failure, features characteristic of TTP.

Distinguishing TTP from atypical HUS is not always possible due to the overlap of symptoms. In the last years a differential diagnosis according to the underlying molecular defect was proposed[126]. In the case of atypical HUS, genetic mutations of genes regulating the complement system and for TTP, deficiency of ADAMTS13 are the proposed patho-mechanisms[111;112].

Congenital TTP is uncommon (2-3% of TTP patients) and it has an autosomal recessive mode of inheritance. Deficiency of ADAMTS13 (levels 5-10% of normal) is due to homozygous or double heterozygous mutations in the *ADAMTS13* gene resulting in constitutional plasma deficiency or in a non-functional protein[41;121]. Until now, more than 70 mutations including missense and nonsense mutations, deletions, insertions, and splice site mutations have been reported[127]. Mutations are not clustered in one gene region, they are spread along the entire length of the gene encoding different protein domains [41]. Single nucleotide polymorphisms of the ADAMTS13 gene, influencing ADAMTS13 secretion and activity have also been described in patients with congenital TTP[121;128]. Congenital TTP generally presents in infancy or childhood, however some patients may develop clinical symptoms of TTP at later age (e.g. during first pregnancy, infections)[129].

Acquired idiopathic TTP is an autoimmune disease with an estimated incidence of ~4 cases/million people[119], occurring mainly in previously healthy individuals. Idiopathic TTP is associated in most of the cases with severe ADAMTS13 deficiency (<10% of normal) and in 60-90% of the patients, inhibitory antibodies that block and reduce ADAMTS13 activity are identified by in vitro functional assays[123]. In a reduced number of cases, the presence of non-inhibitory antibodies was detected by ELISA[130;131]. Non-inhibitory antibodies may be involved in immune complex formation increasing ADAMTS13 clearance or interfering with ADAMTS13 binding to cells or other plasma proteins. Antibodies against ADAMTS13 are predominantly of the IgG and IgM classes[132;133].

Epitope mapping of anti-ADAMTS13 antibodies in TTP patients has demonstrated that the major binding site on ADAMTS13 is located within the cysteine-rich/spacer domains[134;135]. More specifically, amino acids inside the spacer domain (Arg568, Phe592, Arg660, Tyr661 and Tyr665 on the outer surface of the spacer domain), which are directly involved in the interaction with the VWF A2 domain, are the major targeted amino acids by autoantibodies suggesting that autoantibodies may impair the binding of ADAMTS13 to VWF and by consequence inhibit its proteolysis[88;89;136]. However, epitopes on different domains of the ADAMTS13 molecule have also been identified, mostly within the TSP1 2-8 and CUB domains[134;136;137].

Genetic factors also play a role in the etiology of acquired TTP. The presence or reduced levels of the antigens HLA-DRB1*11 and HLA-DRB1*04, respectively was identified as a risk factor for development of acquired TTP[138;139].

## 1.6 Treatment of thrombotic thrombocytopenic purpura

The treatment modalities in patients with TTP differ if the patient suffers from congenital or acquired TTP. Patients with congenital TTP are treated with infusion of normal fresh frozen plasma (FFP) that contains normal levels of ADAMTS13.

Potential relapses in these patients can be prevented or reduced by regular infusions of FFP every 2-3 weeks[117].

The first line therapy for acquired TTP is daily PEX. During the plasmapheresis or PEX procedure, the patient's plasma is extracorporeally separated from the blood cells followed by its replacement by a normal FFP or cryosupernatant and then re-infused together with the blood cells into the blood. The efficacy of PEX therapy has been attributed to the combination of the infusion of normal FFP which supplies ADAMTS13 and the apheresis which removes circulating ULVWF multimers and ADAMTS13 autoantibodies when present[117]. Although PEX is the standard treatment for TTP, it is not safe and adverse events are reported to complicate about 5-12% of the PEX procedures[140]. Immunosuppressive drugs (mainly the steroid methylprednisone) are often added as supportive therapy to improve outcomes.

More recently, the administration of rituximab, a chimeric monoclonal antibody, has been proven to be effective in the treatment of refractory (failure to respond to standard treatment) or relapsing acquired TTP mediated by autoantibodies. Rituximab is an antibody directed against CD20, a surface antigen on B-lymphocytes. Rituximab specifically depletes premature and mature B-cells thus increasing the clearance of antibody-producing cells and by consequence reducing the autoantibody titers[141]. Although there is still limited clinical experience and only few reports outline the advantage of rituximab in patients with TTP, its use appears to be promising and patients seems to benefit through long-lasting remission.

Splenectomy is another therapeutic option indicated in patients suffering of refractory or relapsing TTP. The diagnosis of refractory TTP is considered when incomplete, delayed or no clinical/laboratories responses are obtained with standard treatments within 7 days. Splenectomy has been used with a varying degree of success with its efficacy in preventing relapses remaining controversial[142]. Patients suffering from relapsing TTP seem to have more benefit from the splenectomy than those suffering of refractory TTP[142]. When splenectomy is performed on patients suffering from the relapsing form, it is associated with minimal morbidity and mortality and response rates greater than 80% are achieved[142].

## 1.7 Anti-CD36 antibodies in TTP patients

CD36 (originally identified in platelets as glycoprotein VI) is an integral membrane protein of 471 amino acids that belongs to the class B scavenger receptor family. CD36 is expressed mainly in professional phagocytes, platelets, microvascular endothelium and fat and muscle cells[143]. CD36 has multiple physiologic ligands including oxidized low-density lipoprotein (LDL), phosphatidyl serine (PS) and oxidized PS expressed on the surface of apoptotic cells, long-chain fatty acids and the TSP-1 domains on thrombospondin 1[143]. Based on the wide variety of ligands having diverse and complex functions CD36 could be a critical factor in different diseases such as cancer, atherosclerosis, malaria and insulin resistance[144].

Recent in vitro experiments using recombinant proteins showed that CD36 is able to also bind to ADAMTS13 without inhibiting its activity[61]. The authors suggest that the binding may be mediated via its TSP-1 domains and could be responsible for localizing ADAMTS13 to the surface of endothelial cells[61].

Homozygous or compound heterozygous CD36 deficiency has been reported with variable incidence between different ethnic groups[145]. In addition, a polymorphism in the blood group antigen Nak$^a$ is associated with a selective deficiency of platelet CD36[146]. Interestingly, no clinical symptoms appear to be associated to any type of CD36 deficiency. Patients carrying the platelet CD36 deficiency have no bleeding or thrombotic diatheses but anti-CD36 antibodies were reported in the plasma of some patients due to iso- or alloimmunization against the protein[147].

Interestingly, in about 70% of the patients with acquired TTP, autoantibodies directed against CD36 were detected but their pathological or clinical significance was not investigated[148-150]. The presence of autoantibodies against CD36 has also been described in patients suffering from autoimmune diseases such as SLE[151] and antiphospholipid syndrome[152]. More recently, Rock et al[153] described the concomitant presence of anti-CD36 and anti-ADAMTS13 antibodies in 16/35 patients analyzed, suggesting a possible pathogenic role of these antibodies in TTP.

## 2- AIM OF THE THESIS

The main goal of the thesis was to characterize the antibody response against the metalloprotease ADAMTS13 in patients suffering from acquired thrombotic thrombocytopenic purpura (TTP). Our group was the first to describe the presence of anti-ADAMTS13 IgG and IgM antibodies in TTP patients. These findings prompted a further characterization of the immune response in a cohort of adult patients with acute acquired TTP to better understand the patho-mechanism leading to acquired TTP. In addition, we attempted to investigate possible prognostic or predictive marker/s that could help to identify patients at risk of recurrence or fatal outcome.

## DESIGN OF THE RESEARCH STUDY

The following aspects shall be investigated in a cohort of 76 patients diagnosed with acute acquired TTP:

- *Evaluation of ADAMTS13-specific activity, functional inhibitors and antigen levels.*
  The quantification of these parameters will be performed using standard assays.
- *Detection of total IgG, IgG subclasses, IgM, IgA and IgE anti-ADAMTS13 antibodies.*
  The detection of IgG and IgM antibodies in plasma will be performed using a pre-established in-house enzyme-linked immunosorbent assay (ELISA). For detection of IgG subclasses, IgA and IgE antibodies, specific ELISA systems will be established.
- *Detection of circulating ADAMTS13-anti-ADAMTS13 antibody immune complexes (IC).*
  For detection of ADAMTS13-specific IC in plasma two different assays will be developed. (1) A co-immunoprecipitation of plasma ADAMTS13 with IgG, IgM, and IgA antibodies. (2) ELISA-based systems to detect and characterize the immunoglobulin type and subclass involved in the IC formation.
- *Detection of anti-CD36 antibodies.*
  For detection of anti-CD36 antibodies in plasma a specific ELISA will be established.
- *Correlation of the different parameters evaluated with the clinical outcome of the patients*

The different parameters evaluated will be correlated with the clinical outcome of the patients using standard statistical tests and software.

# 3- METHODOLOGY

## 3.1 Patients

### 3.1.1 Plasma samples

Frozen plasma samples from TTP patients were obtained from three European Reference Centers: the Central Hematology Laboratory, University of Bern, Switzerland (Center 1), Service d'Hematologie biologique, Hôspital Antoine Béclère, Paris, France (Center 2) and Department of Medicine 1, Medical University of Vienna, Vienna, Austria (Center 3). Patients were enrolled after giving consent according to The Declaration of Helsinki. This study was approved by the institutional review board.

Plasma samples from healthy donors were collected at plasma collection centers of Baxter Innovations in Austria.

### 3.1.2 Sample collection

Before any therapeutical treatment was initiated, venous blood samples were collected into tubes containing 3.8% (w/v) sodium citrate and platelet-poor plasma was obtained by centrifugation at 2500 x g for 15 minutes. Plasma aliquots were stored at $-80°C$ until tested. For one patient, daily plasma samples (time course samples during 2 months follow-up (death)) were collected before initiation of therapeutic PEX in which patient' plasma is replaced by normal fresh frozen plasma.

### 3.1.3 Inclusion criteria

Patients had to meet the following inclusion criteria: (i) presence of microangiopathic hemolytic anemia (hemoglobin level <12 g/dL), direct antiglobulin test negative, at least 2 schistocytes per high-power field in the peripheral blood smear, LDH levels >450 IU/L and undetectable serum haptoglobin; (ii) thrombocytopenia (platelet count <150 x 10$^9$/L); (iii) severely reduced (<10%) plasma ADAMTS13 activity levels. Fever, neurological symptoms or renal failure were not obligatory.

### 3.1.4 Clinical definition

Idiopathic TTP was defined as TTP occurring in patients with no apparent preexisting disease. Patients are described as having secondary TTP if other conditions are identified that may cause thrombotic microangiopathy such as pregnancy, other autoimmune diseases, HIV infection and cancer. Remission was defined as a normal platelet count (>150 x 109/L) and no plasma exchange treatment for 30 consecutive days (day 1 of remission) or more. Relapse or recurrence was defined as the reappearance of clinical manifestation and/or laboratory data compatible with TTP after remission had been achieved. Refractory TTP is considered when incomplete, delayed or no clinical and laboratories responses are obtained with standard treatments within 7 days.

## 3.2 Measurement of the ADAMTS13 activity and inhibitor

## 3.2.1 Measurement of the ADAMTS13 activity

The measurements of residual ADAMTS13 activity (ADAMTS13:Ac) and anti-ADAMTS13 inhibitory activity in patients´ plasma were carried out in the participant centers at the moment when the patient was admitted to the hospital.

In Center 1, the ADAMTS13 activity and inhibitor was tested according to Studt *et al*[154] using a quantitative immunoblotting assay and in Center 2 according to Veyradier *et al*[155] using a two-site ELISA assay. Both methods measure ADAMTS13 activity under static conditions, employing multimeric/full-length VWF as substrate and indirect quantification of the VWF cleavage products by immunoblotting or ELISA. Both methods have similar sensitivities[105].

## 3.2.2 Measurement of the ADAMTS13 activity by FRETS-VWF73 assay

Samples received from Center 3 were tested in our laboratory using the FRETS-VWF73 assay performed essentially as described[100] with minor modifications. Plasma samples were diluted 1 to 25 in assay buffer (5 mM Bis-Tris, 25 mM CaCl2, 0.005% v/v Tween 20, pH 6.0) supplemented with a protease inhibitor cocktail (Sigma, St. Louis, MO, USA) in a final concentration of 2 µL/ 100 µL of reaction buffer and 2% v/v heat-inactivated pooled normal human plasma (NHP) (George King Bio-Medical, Overland Park, KS, USA) to correct for a plasma matrix effect in the dilution. The heat-inactivation of the plasmas was achieved by incubating the plasma at 56°C for 30 min followed by 15 min of centrifugation at 15000 x g. A calibration curve was made diluting a pooled NHP (George King Bio-Medical) 1 to 25 and by serial dilutions in a ratio of 3 to 4 (75%), 1 to 2 (50%), 1 to 4 (25%), 1 to 8 (12.5%), 1 to 16 (6.25%) and 1 to 32 (3.12%) in supplemented assay buffer. The FRETS-VWF73 substrate (Peptide Institute Inc., Osaka, Japan) was re-suspended in

25% v/v dimethylsulfoxide, leading to 100 μM FRETS-VWF73 stock solution and subsequently diluted to a final concentration of 1.67 μM in assay buffer without supplementation. 100 μL/well of each diluted plasma sample or standard was added to a 96-well white plate (Costar, Corning Inc., NY, USA) followed by the addition of 100 μL/well FRETS-VWF73 substrate. The fluorescence was measured at 37°C every 5 min for 90 min in a SAFIRE II reader (Tecan, Zürich, Switzerland) equipped with a 340 nm excitation filter and 440 nm emission filter. The reaction rate was calculated by linear regression analysis of fluorescence over time and compared with that of a pooled NHP used as calibration curve.

## 3.2.3 Anti-ADAMTS13 inhibitor activity assay

The ADAMTS13 functional inhibitor titers were measured according to the Bethesda method originally described for anti-factor VIII antibodies[104]. Briefly, patient' plasma and pooled NHP were heat-inactivated (as described in chapter 3.2.2) to inactivate any endogenous ADAMTS13 activity. Afterwards, a mixture of equal volumes of heat-inactivated patient' plasma and pooled NHP as well as a control mixture made of buffer and pooled NHP were incubated for 2 hours at 37°C. After incubation, the residual ADAMTS13:Ac in both mixtures was assayed. The residual ADAMTS13:Ac is defined as the percentage between the residual ADAMTS13:Ac of the patient' mixture compared with the control mixture. A patient was considered to have inhibitors of ADAMTS13 if the residual ADAMTS13:Ac in the patient' mixture was less than 75% of the control mixture. When the residual ADAMTS13:Ac of the mixture with the undiluted sample was below 25%, samples were retested by diluting until a residual ADAMTS13:Ac between 25% and 75% was obtained. The inhibitor titers are expressed in Bethesda Units per milliliter (BU/mL) and one BU is defined as the amount of inhibitor that results in 50% residual ADAMTS13:Ac. The inhibitor titer of the patient' plasma is read from a semi-logarithmic plot representing the correlation between residual ADAMTS13:Ac (logarithmic) and the inhibitor titer in BU/mL (linear). The regression line is defined by 100% residual ADAMTS13:Ac when no inhibitor is present (0 BU/mL) and 50% residual ADAMTS13:Ac when 1 BU/mL inhibitor is present.

The procedure described above was followed by all the participant Centers with a minor modification in the incubation time done by Center 2 (30 min at room temperature (RT) instead of 2 hours at 37°C). The residual ADAMTS13:Ac was measured by the FRETS-VWF73 assay or the immunoblotting assay[154] (Center 1) or by ELISA[155] (Center 2).

There was a difference in the expression of inhibitor titers between Centers. Center 1 reported the exact inhibitor titers when the BU/mL were up to 2. When the residual ADAMTS13:Ac was between 11% and 25% (titers greater than 2 BU/mL), titers were reported as >2 BU/mL. When the residual ADAMTS13:Ac was equal or less than 10%, titers are reported as >>2 BU/mL. Center 2 expressed the titers semi-quantitatively; they were arbitrarily defined as high, medium or low for a residual ADAMTS13:Ac less than 10% in a 1:1, 2:1 or 3:1 volume/volume mixture of patient and pooled NHP, respectively.

Due to these differences in the expression of the ADAMTS13 functional inhibitor titers between Centers 1 and 2, a harmonization of the titer results was arbitrarily done to express them by a single measure. Inhibitor titers from Center 1 were assigned as low, medium or high when the BU were up to 2 BU/mL, >2 BU/mL and >>2 BU/mL, respectively.

## 3.3 Measurement of ADAMTS13 protein (antigen) levels

ADAMTS13 antigen (ADAMTS13:Ag) levels were analyzed in patients' plasma by ELISA according to Rieger *et al*[51]. Microtiter plates (Nunc-Immuno Maxisorp, Roskilde, Denmark) were coated with 100 µL/well of a polyclonal rabbit anti-human ADAMTS13 IgG (2 µg/mL; Baxter Innovations, Vienna, Austria) in 0.1 M bicarbonate solution, pH 9.6 for 5 hours at RT. The non-specific binding sites were blocked with 0.5% w/v non-fat dry milk (Blotting Grade Blocker Non-Fat Dry Milk, Bio-Rad Laboratories, CA, USA) diluted into phosphate-buffered saline (PBS), pH 7.4, containing 0.1% v/v Tween-20 (Biorad) (PBS-T). Plasma and standard samples (100 µL/well) were incubated overnight at RT. Plates were washed and incubated with 100 µL/well of a horseradish peroxidase (HRP)-conjugated polyclonal rabbit anti-human ADAMTS13 IgG (Baxter) at 20 ng/mL and developed using 100 µL/well of the chromogenic 3,3',5,5'-tetra-methylbenzidine substrate (TMB; Sure Blue™ TMB Microwell Peroxidase Substrate, KPL, Maryland, USA). The color reaction was stopped by the addition of 50 µL/well of 1 N HCl and the absorbance was read at 450 nm with a reference filter of 620 nm on an iEMS microplate reader (Labsystems, Helsinki, Finland). Between each step, the plates were washed with PBS-T in an auto strip washer (Elx50 Bio-Tek instruments, Germany).

ADAMTS13:Ag levels in the samples were calculated extrapolating the corresponding OD value from a standard curve using purified recombinant ADAMTS13 (rADAMTS13, Baxter Innovations) diluted to final concentrations of 20, 10, 5, 2.5, 1.25, 0.625 and 0.5 ng/mL in ADAMTS13-depleted human plasma (Baxter Innovations). The reference interval for the ELISA (calculated with 100 individual healthy donors) was 740–1420 ng ADAMTS13/mL and the limit of quantification was 62.5 ng ADAMTS13/mL. Samples with antigen levels under the limit of quantification were expressed as <62.5 ng ADAMTS13/mL.

## 3.4 Detection of anti-ADAMTS13 antibodies

### 3.4.1 ELISA to detect total IgG, IgG subclass, IgM, IgA and IgE anti-ADAMTS13 antibodies

The presence of total IgG (IgGtot) and IgG subclasses, IgM, IgA and IgE anti-ADAMTS13 antibodies in patient plasmas was tested by ELISA as described[132] with minor modifications. Microtiter plates (Nunc) were coated with an anti-His tag antibody (2 µg/mL; Penta-His, Qiagen, Hilden, Germany) by overnight incubation at 4°C. The non-specific binding sites were blocked with PBS containing 2% w/v bovine serum albumin (BSA, Sigma) (PBS-BSA) and thereafter, 100µL/well recombinant His-tagged ADAMTS13 (Baxter Innovations) was added in a concentration of 2 µg/mL diluted in PBS-BSA. Diluted patients' plasma and negative controls (pooled NHP of 30 healthy donors, Baxter Innovations) were incubated overnight at 4°C. Bound antibodies were detected using an alkaline-phosphatase (AP)-conjugated goat anti-human IgG, IgM, IgA or IgE antibody (Sigma) or mouse monoclonal anti-human IgG1, IgG2, IgG3 or IgG4 antibodies (Zymed Laboratories, San Francisco, CA, USA). Finally, the enzyme substrate p-nitrophenylphosphate (pNPP; Sigma) was added, and the absorbance was read at 405 nm with a reference filter of 620 nm on a microplate reader (Labsystems). Between each step, the plates were washed with PBS-T in an auto strip washer (Bio-Tek instruments).

### 3.4.2 Cross-reactivity assay

The specificity in the detection of the AP-conjugated mouse monoclonal anti-human IgG1-IgG4 and the goat anti-human IgA and IgE antibodies used in the ELISAs was tested in an ELISA-based cross-reactivity assay. Briefly, microtiter plates (Nunc) were coated with 100 µL/well of purified human IgG1-4, IgM, IgA and IgE (Sigma) diluted in a concentration range between 4 and 0.1 µg/mL using PBS. After overnight incubation at 4°C, the plates were washed and incubated with 100 µL/well of an AP-conjugated goat anti-human IgA or IgE antibody (Sigma) or monoclonal AP-conjugated mouse anti-human IgG1, IgG2, IgG3 and IgG4 antibodies (Zymed). The enzyme substrate pNPP (Sigma) was added, and the absorbance was read at 405 nm with a reference filter of 620 nm on a microplate reader (Labsystems). No cross-reactivity was observed at any concentration with any class or subclass of antibodies analyzed.

### 3.4.3 Data analysis and cut-off calculations

IgGtot and IgG subclass, IgM, IgA and IgE anti-ADAMTS13 antibodies detected by the ELISA described in chapter 3.4.1 were expressed as antibody titers. For calculation of the anti-ADAMTS13 antibody titers, the ELISA read out (optical density, OD) from 100 healthy donors diluted in a range between 1 to 20 up to 1 to 6400 was used to calculate the ratio of sample OD to background OD for each sample at each dilution. As background OD the signal derived from a pooled NHP was used. To achieve an approximate normal distribution, the OD ratio values of the 100 control plasmas were transformed by the function $y=\log(1+\log(x))$. Normal distribution was assessed by quantile-quantile plots and Shapiro-Wilk tests. The means and standard deviations of the resulting 100 ratios were calculated. The thresholds for each dilution were obtained by back-transformation of the means plus two standard deviations of the transformed data. Samples with ratios below or above the cut-off levels were judged as negative or positive, respectively. When a sample was judged positive, sample dilutions were compared with the corresponding cut-off value and the last dilution above the cut–off value was taken as positive.

For the IgG subclass ELISA, the OD values were additionally normalized by the corresponding normalization factor and calculated as described below.

### 3.4.4 Quantification and normalization of the absorbances measured in the IgG subclass ELISA

An ELISA with subclass-specific antibodies was used to estimate the relative amount of the different IgG subclasses, first because of the absence of a true standard, and second because of the differences in the development time between the IgG subclasses due to differences in the detection sensitivities of the secondary antibodies used. To minimize these differences, the relative OD values of the IgG subclass ELISA were compared under standardized conditions.

Each IgG subclass (purified human IgG1-IgG4, Sigma) was coated on an ELISA plate in a concentration range of 0.125 to 1 µg/mL and the time-dependent OD signal generated was analyzed. The corresponding OD values generated were recorded every 5 min up to 75 min, and plotted against time. Slopes for each concentration and subclass were calculated. The corresponding means ± standard deviations of the slopes from 4 independent experiments were plotted and analyzed by linear regression for each individual IgG subclass. The regression parameters obtained were used to calculate the OD values of each subclass at a coating concentration of 0.5 µg/mL (linear range). The OD value of IgG4 was set to "1", resulting in normalization factors for IgG1, IgG2 and IgG3 of 9, 0.7 and 0.4, as compared with IgG4. Coating efficiency was evaluated in each experiment by ELISA using an AP-conjugated goat anti-human lambda light chain antibody (Sigma) to ensure uniform IgG1-IgG4 concentrations.

The calculated normalization factors were used to normalize the OD values in patients with more than one IgG subclass of anti-ADAMTS13 antibodies. Samples were normalized by multiplying the OD values corresponding to each positive subclass by the corresponding calculated normalization factor. With this approach, an estimate of the relative contributions of the different IgG subclasses to the total anti-ADAMTS13 IgG in patient plasma was obtained. Without the normalization procedure, IgG1 levels would have been underestimated as compared to IgG2, IgG3 and IgG4 levels. Samples with normalized OD values above the linear range were excluded (six patients) from analyses.

Positive normalized OD values of each subclass were summed up ($IgG_{sum}$, total absorbance) and the proportion of each individual subclass was calculated as a percentage of the total absorbance (assumed to be 100%) to obtain the IgG subclass percentage distribution in a single patient.

### 3.4.5 Competitive inhibition of antibody binding with recombinant ADAMTS13

To ensure specificity of the anti-ADAMTS13 antibody detection, competitive inhibition experiments with rADAMTS13 in solution were carried out. Diluted patient and pooled NHP plasmas were pre-incubated with 100 µg/mL of purified rADAMTS13 at 37°C for 2 hours to allow binding of ADAMTS13-specific antibodies to rADAMTS13 in solution. Afterwards, the binding of anti-ADAMTS13 antibodies was assayed by the ELISA as described above (chapter 3.4.1). As negative control, plasma samples were pre-incubated with BSA (100 µg/mL). A sample was judged as positive when addition of rADAMTS13 decreased the antibody binding by at least 30% when compared to the decrease of the negative control.

## 3.5 Detection of IgG anti-ADAMTS13 antibodies by a commercial ELISA kit

The measurement of IgG anti-ADAMTS13 antibodies was also performed using a commercially available kit (TECHNOZYM ADAMTS-13 INH; Technoclone GmbH, Vienna, Austria) according to the manufacturer´s instructions. Briefly, 100 µL/well of diluted plasma samples or calibrators were added to wells coated with rADAMTS13 and incubated for 1 hour at RT. Thereafter, 100 µL/well of a HRP-conjugated anti-human IgG were added followed by 100 µL/well of the chromogenic substrate TMB. The color reaction was stopped by the addition of 1.9 M $H_2SO_4$ and the absorbance was measured at 450 nm with a reference filter of 620 nm on a microplate reader (Labsystems).

The antibody titers of a sample were obtained by extrapolating from the corresponding OD value of a standard curve using standards provided with the kit in concentrations ranging between 0.8-98.8 U/mL of anti-ADAMTS13 antibodies. Standards are calibrated against a plasma with a very high titer of IgG anti-ADAMST13. A 1 to 200 dilution of this reference plasma is defined to contain an antibody concentration of 100 U/mL (arbitrary units).

The positive cut-off value of the assay is 15 U/mL, samples with results between 12-15 U/mL are judged as borderline and samples with values below 12 U/mL are judged as negative.

## 3.6 Detection of circulating immune complexes by co-immunoprecipitation and Western blotting

Patient plasma (200 µL) was incubated with 100 µL protein G Sepharose (Protein G HP SpinTrap$^{TM}$ columns, GE Healthcare, Buckinghamshire, England) or anti-IgA or anti-IgM specific affinity matrixes (BAC CaptureSelect, Naarden, The Netherlands) for 30 min (IgG) and 120 min, respectively at RT on a rotator. The immunoprecipitated IgG-, IgA-, or IgM containing material was washed 6 times with binding buffer (20 mM sodium phosphate, 150 mM NaCl; pH 7.0) and the antigen-antibody complexes were eluted from the beads by adding sample loading buffer (Thermo, Rockford, IL, USA) and heating at 95°C for 10 min. The resulting supernatants were loaded on a 4–12% gradient tris-glycine SDS polyacrylamide pre-cast gel (Invitrogen, Caramillo, CA, USA) and subjected to electrophoresis under reducing conditions. The separated proteins were transferred to a polyvinyldifluoride membrane using an iBlot® Dry Blotting System (Invitrogen), and ADAMTS13 was detected with an affinity-purified polyclonal rabbit IgG anti-human ADAMTS13 antibody (1 µg/mL; Baxter Innovations) in combination with a HRP-conjugated goat anti-rabbit IgG (27 ng/mL; Jackson Immunoresearch, West Grove, PA, USA) and addition of a chemiluminescent substrate (Thermo). Immunoreactive bands were visualized with the Fusion FX7 image system (Vilber Lourmat, Germany). The ADAMTS13 luminograms were scanned and the relative amount of immune complexes (ICs; expressed in arbitrary units (AU)) was quantified by densitometry using the BIO-1D software (Vilber Lourmat) and rADAMTS13 (1 ng) as standard.

To evaluate for unspecific binding to the matrix, human serum albumin (HSA) in a final concentration of 50 µg/mL was spiked with 2 µg/mL rADAMTS13 and processed as the plasma samples. For the anti-IgA matrix, a minimal unspecific binding was observed with the negative controls. In this case, the mean background signal generated by the pooled NHP and ADAMTS13-spiked samples was subtracted from the signal of the plasma samples.

## 3.7 Detection of circulating immune complexes by ELISA

Microtiter plates (Nunc) were coated with 100 µL/well of a polyclonal rabbit anti-human ADAMTS13 IgG (2 µg/mL; Baxter Innovations) in 0.05 M carbonate-bicarbonate buffer, pH 9.6 by overnight incubation at 4°C. The non-specific binding sites were blocked with 0.5% w/v non-fat dry milk (Bio-Rad) diluted into PBS-T buffer. A 100 µL/well of diluted patient and normal plasmas (dilution range: 1 to 20, 1 to 50 and 1 to 100) were incubated overnight at 4°C. Thereafter, plates were washed and incubated with 100 µL/well of an AP-conjugated goat anti-human IgA (Sigma) or mouse monoclonal anti-human IgG1, IgG2, IgG3 and IgG4 antibodies (Zymed Laboratories). Finally, the enzyme substrate 5-bromo-4-chloro-3-indoyl phosphate (BCIP) (KPL) was added, and the absorbance was read at 620 nm on an iEMS microplate reader (Labsystems). Between each step, the plates were washed with PBS-T in an auto strip washer (Elx50 Bio-Tek instruments).

For cut-off calculation, 60 healthy donors diluted in the same range as the samples were used to calculate the ratio of sample OD to background OD (signal derived from a pooled NHP). Normal distribution was assessed by the Shapiro-Wilk test and the means plus three standard deviations of the resulting 60 ratios were calculated for each dilution. Samples with ratios below or above the cut-off levels were judged as negative or positive, respectively.

### 3.7.1 Detection of complement fixing immune complexes by C1q binding ELISA

Complement fixing immune complexes (ICs) were analyzed using a C1q binding ELISA kit (Bühlmann Laboratories, Schönenbuch, Switzerland) according to the manufacturer's instructions. Briefly, patient plasma, calibrators and controls were incubated with human C1q adsorbed on a microtiter plate. After incubation, AP-conjugated Protein A was added, followed by the enzyme substrate pNPP. The color reaction was stopped after 30 min of incubation by the addition of 1 N NaOH and the absorbance was measured at 450 nm with a reference filter of 620 nm on a microplate reader (Labsystems).

The concentration of ICs present in the plasma samples was determined by extrapolating the corresponding OD value to a standard curve using standards provided with the kit. Results were expressed as heat aggregated human gamma globulin equivalents per mL (µg Eq/mL). The negative cut-off value of the assay is 3.2 µg Eq/mL, samples between 3.2-5.0 µg Eq/mL are judged as borderline and samples with values above 5.0 µg Eq/mL are judged as positive.

### 3.7.2 Competitive inhibition of the binding of human IgG4 to rabbit anti-ADAMTS13 antibody

To confirm unspecific binding of human IgG4 to rabbit anti-ADAMTS13 antibody coated on the plate, a competitive inhibition experiment was performed. Diluted normal plasma (dilution range: 1 to 20, 1 to 50, 1 to 100, 1 to 200, 1 to 400 and 1 to 800) was pre-incubated with 11 µg/mL monoclonal mouse anti-human IgG4 antibody (Sigma) at 37°C for 30 min. After incubation, the binding of human IgG4 was assayed by ELISA as described in chapter 3.7. As negative control, diluted plasma samples were pre-incubated with 11 µg/mL of BSA diluted in PBS.

### 3.7.3 Binding of rabbit IgG to human antibodies

Microtiter plates (Nunc) were coated by overnight incubation at 4°C with 100 µL/well of purified human IgG1-4 (Sigma), IgM (Sigma) and IgA (Calbiochem, Darmstadt, Germany) in a concentration of 4 µg/mL diluted in 0.05 M carbonate-bicarbonate buffer, pH 9.6. The non-specific binding sites were blocked with 0.5% non-fat dry milk (Bio-Rad) diluted in PBS-T buffer. Thereafter, plates were washed and incubated with 100 µL/well of HRP-conjugated rabbit IgG (whole molecule) or rabbit IgG Fc fragment or rabbit IgG F(ab)2 fragment (Alpha Diagnostic, San Antonio, TX, USA), in a concentration range between 1 and 4 µg/mL. After 4 hours of incubation, plates were developed with TMB substrate (KPL) and the color reaction was stopped by the addition of 1 N HCl. The absorbance was read at 450 nm with a reference filter of 620 nm on a microplate reader (Labsystems). Between each step, the plates were washed with PBS-T in an auto strip washer (Bio-Tek instruments).

## 3.8 Detection of anti-CD36 antibodies by ELISA

Microtiter plates (Half area, high binding; Costar, Corning Inc., NY, USA) were coated with 50 µL/well of recombinant full-length CD36 (1.5 µg/mL; Origene, Rockville, USA) diluted in 0.05 M carbonate-bicarbonate buffer, pH 9.6 by overnight incubation at 4°C. The non-specific binding sites were blocked with Protein-Free blocking buffer (Thermo). Afterwards, 50 µL/well of patient and normal plasmas (diluted 1 to 50 in LowCross buffer (Candor Bioscience, Weissensberg, Germany) were added and incubated for additional 3 hours at RT. Plates were washed and incubated for 90 min at RT with 50 µL/well of biotin-conjugated goat anti-human IgG antibody (Rockland Immunochemicals, Gilbersville, PA, USA) at 10 ng/mL in LowCross buffer followed by the addition of streptavidin-peroxidase polymer conjugate (Sigma) diluted 1 to 5000 in PBS. Plates were developed by the addition of 50 µL/well of the TMB substrate (KPL) and the color reaction stopped with 50 µL/well of 1 N HCl. Absorbance was read at 450 nm with a reference filter of 620 nm on a microplate reader (Labsystems). Between each step, the plates were washed with PBS-T in an auto strip washer (Bio-Tek instruments).

As a positive ELISA control, a monoclonal rat anti-human CD36 antibody (R&D Systems, Minneapolis, MN, USA) was tested in a concentration range between 0 and 60 ng/mL and detected with HRP-conjugated rabbit anti-rat IgG (whole molecule, 100ng/mL, Sigma).

For cut-off calculation, 60 healthy donors were used to calculate the ratio of sample OD to background OD (signal derived from a pooled NHP). Normal distribution was assessed by the Shapiro-Wilk test after log-transformation of the data and the means and standard deviations of the resulting 60 ratios were calculated. The thresholds for each dilution were obtained by back-transformation of the means plus three standard deviations of the transformed data. Samples with ratios below or above the cut-off levels were judged as negative or positive, respectively.

To ensure that the detected anti-CD36 antibodies are specific, positive samples were subjected to competitive inhibition using an excess of rCD36 (11 µg/mL) in solution. Following pre-incubation with soluble rCD36 at 37°C for 2 hours, patient and pooled NHP plasma samples were assayed for anti-CD36 antibodies by the ELISA as described above.

## 3.9 Statistical analysis

Statistical analyses were done with SigmaStat version 3.5 (Systat Software, San Jose, CA, USA). Demographic and clinical data are presented as the median and the interquartile range (IQR). Cut-off values for the different established ELISAs were calculated as described in the corresponding chapter. The statistical significance of the differences between OD ratios of healthy donors and TTP patients were assessed by the Mann-Whitney rank sum test. The statistical significance of the differences between medians of IgG1 and IgG4 values were assessed by the Mann-Whitney rank sum test and the correlation by the Spearman rank test. To assess the strength of the relation between IgG4 levels and recurrence, 40 patients were divided into three groups according to clinical outcome. The first group comprised 18 patients who had experienced only a single TTP event, the second comprised nine patients who relapsed during the 36 months of follow-up and the third comprised 13 patients who had had relapse(s), five of whom had had no further relapses during follow-up and eight of whom were lost to follow-up after the acute relapsing event. Deceased patients, patients lost to follow-up after the first TTP event and patients with IgG4 OD values above the linear range were excluded from this analysis (18 patients). *P*-values less than 0.05 were considered to be statistically significant.

# 4- RESULTS

## 4.1 Demographic and clinical features of the patients enrolled

Seventy-six adult patients diagnosed with acute acquired TTP were included in the study. All of them met the inclusion criteria described in chapter 3.1.3. Demographic, clinical and standard biological features of the 76 patients enrolled are summarized in Table 1. The median age was 37 year-old (range 16-75) and the sex ratio was 2F/1M (50 women and 26 men). Sixty-three had idiopathic TTP and thirteen had TTP associated with pregnancy ($n=6$), the postpartum state ($n=1$), psoriasis ($n=1$), antiphospholipid syndrome ($n=1$), SLE ($n=1$), renal disease ($n=2$) or cancer ($n=1$).

**Table 1. Demographic and clinical features of the patients with acute acquired thrombotic thrombocytopenic purpura (TTP) included in the study**

| | |
|---|---|
| Sex, F/M | 50/26 |
| Median age, years (range) | 37 (16-75) |
| Median platelet count, $x10^9 L^{-1}$ (range) | 15 (2-96) |
| Median hemoglobin levels, g/dL (range)* | 9.6 (4.2-14.7) |
| No of patients / total | |
|     Idiopathic TTP | 63/76 |
|     TTP with associated conditions | 13/76 |
|     First episode | 57/76 |
|     Relapse | 19/76 |
| Renal involvement[#] | 9/68 |
| Neurological symptoms[#] | 27/68 |

\* data were not available for 8 patients
[#] data were not available for 17 patients

Renal involvement was considered when plasmatic creatinine values were above 120 µmol/L. Neurological involvement included: aphasia, headache, confusion, paresthesia, altered mental status and seizure.

Fifty-seven patients were analyzed during the first acute episode of TTP and 19 during relapse. Four of the 57 (7%) patients analyzed during the first episode died of acute multivisceral thrombotic microangiopathy, 10 patients were lost to follow-up and 12/43 who achieved clinical remission, relapsed during a minimum of 48-months follow-up (follow-up performed in a range of 48 to 109 months). The 19 patients studied during an acute relapse had a documented positive history of TTP with at least one previous TTP episode. Seven of the 19 patients were included in the 48-months follow-up and they had no new relapses and 12/19 patients were lost to follow-up.

At inclusion during the acute episode, anemia (hemoglobin median levels 9.6 g/dL; range 4.2–14.7 g/dL; data available only for 59/76 patients) and thrombocytopenia (median $15 \times 10^9$/L; range $2$-$96 \times 10^9$/L) were present in the patients. Neurologic symptoms including headache, altered mental status, aphasia, paresthesia, transitory ischemic attack or convulsions were observed in 27/68 (40%) patients. Renal involvement, considered when plasmatic creatinine values were higher than 200 µmol/L, was present only in 9/68 (13%) patients whereas the mean creatinine level was $101 \pm 31$ µmol/L in the remaining 59 patients. For 8 patients, the neurological and renal data were not available.

## 4.2 ADAMTS13 activity, functional ADAMTS13 inhibitor and ADAMTS13 antigen levels in patients with acquired TTP

As a result of our inclusion criteria, all patients ($n$=76) had ADAMTS13:Ac values <10%. A functional inhibitor was found in 69/76 (91%) patients; with 26 patients having a low, 23 patients a medium and 20 patients a high titer. In 7 (9%) patients a functional inhibitor was not detected by the assays used at the respective reference center.

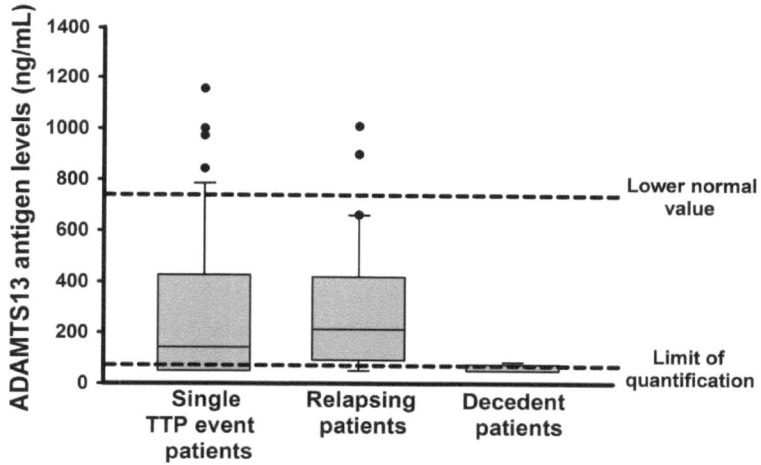

**Figure 4. ADAMTS13 antigen levels in patients with acquired TTP.**
Box plot of the distribution of the ADAMTS13 antigen levels in 76 patients with acute acquired TTP. Patients are divided into 3 categories according to the clinical outcome. The lower normal value (740 ng/mL) and the limit of quantification (<65 ng/mL) are indicated by dashed lines. The bottom, median and top lines of the box mark the $25^{th}$, $50^{th}$, and $75^{th}$ percentiles, respectively. The vertical line shows the range of values comprised between the $5^{th}$ and $95^{th}$ percentiles and the dots represent outlier values.

Analysis of ADAMTS13:Ag levels in TTP patients showed a variable distribution similar to earlier findings[51]. Eighteen patients had undetectable levels (<65 ng/mL), 10 patients had severely reduced antigen levels (65-100 ng/mL), 42 patients had reduced levels (100-740 ng/mL) and 6 patients had normal levels. There were no differences when the antigen levels between patients with single or relapsing TTP events were compared (Fig. 4). Three of the four deceased patients had undetectable antigen levels and the fourth one a borderline level (83 ng/mL) (Fig. 4).

## 4.3 Anti-ADAMTS13 antibody profile in patients with acquired TTP

To investigate the presence of anti-ADAMTS13 antibodies, in-house ELISA assays were employed. These ELISAs use immobilized recombinant ADAMTS13 and bound plasma antibodies are visualized by means of specific secondary, enzyme-labeled antibodies.

For detection of IgG and IgM anti-ADAMTS13 antibodies, previously established in-house ELISA assays were used[132]. For detection of IgA, IgE and IgG subclasses, new ELISA assays were developed introducing a single modification to the pre-established ELISA at the level of the secondary antibody.

### 4.3.1 Anti-ADAMTS13 antibody profile in the acute episode

Analysis of the anti-ADAMTS13 antibody profile in the acute episode showed the presence of anti-ADAMTS13 antibodies in 71/76 (93%) patients.

IgG anti-ADAMTS13 antibodies were detected by our in-house ELISA in 52/76 TTP patients. In patients whose anti-ADAMTS13 IgG titers were lower than the detection limit of our ELISA (IgG negative, 18 patients), plasma samples were retested for anti-ADAMTS13 IgG antibodies using a commercial kit with improved sensitivity due to the use of a horseradish peroxidase-conjugated secondary antibody instead of an alkaline-phosphatase-conjugated one. Using this kit, 12/18 patients tested positive for IgG anti-ADAMTS13 antibodies and 6 patients were confirmed negative.

Taking together the results of both ELISA assays (in-house and commercial), 70/76 (92%) patients with acute TTP had a specific IgG against ADAMTS13 with titers ranging from 20 to 6400 (Fig. 5).

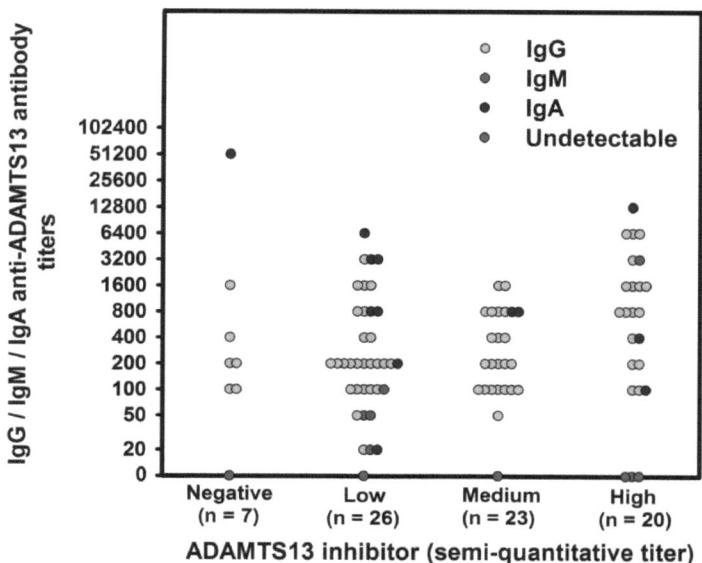

**Figure 5. ADAMTS13 inhibitor and anti-ADAMTS13 IgG/IgM/IgA antibodies in patients with acquired TTP.**

Seventy-six patients with acute acquired TTP were analyzed for the presence of ADAMTS13 inhibitor and the different classes of anti-ADAMTS13 antibodies. Patients are grouped in 4 categories according to their ADAMTS13 inhibitor titers (semi-quantitative): negative (7 patients), low (26 patients), medium (23 patients) and high (20 patients). Each patient is represented by a symbol. Gray circles are for patients with positive IgG, green circles for IgM, blue circles for IgA and red circles for patients with no detectable IgG/IgM/IgA (undetectable). Only positive patients are depicted for IgM and IgA antibodies.

IgM and IgA classes of anti-ADAMTS13 antibodies were investigated in addition to the IgG class. Low titers (ranging from 20-100 with exception of one patient with 3200) of IgM anti-ADAMTS13 antibodies were detected in 5/76 (7%) patients (Fig. 5). IgA anti-ADAMTS13 antibodies were found in 13/75 (17%) patients with variable titers from 200 to 51200 (Fig. 5). In one patient, the IgA anti-ADAMTS13 antibody titer could not be determined due to the lack of a sufficient amount of plasma.

A trend toward increasing inhibiting activity with increasing anti-ADAMTS13 titers was observed, especially in those patients positive for more than one class of antibodies (Fig. 5).

Isolated IgG anti-ADAMTS13 antibodies were detected in 57 patients. IgM was not detected alone and only one patient had low titer of IgA antibodies. The combination of IgG and IgM was detected in 2 patients, the combination of IgG and IgA in 8 patients and the combination of the 3 classes of antibodies in 3 patients. Taken together, 71 out of 76 (93%) patients tested positive for anti-ADAMTS13 antibodies.

The presence of non inhibitory antibodies was detected in 6 out of 7 patients with no measurable functional inhibitor (Fig. 5). Five patients tested positive only for IgG antibodies and the sixth one for IgG in combination with high IgA antibodies. One patient tested negative for both ADAMTS13 functional inhibitor and classes (IgG, IgM or IgA) of anti-ADAMTS13 antibodies. The overall prevalence of non inhibitory antibodies in this study was 8%.

An interesting finding is that the plasma from 4 patients inhibited ADAMTS13 activity in the absence of any detectable class (IgG, IgM or IgA) of anti-ADAMTS13 antibodies.

## 4.3.2 Correlation between ADAMTS13 antibodies at presentation and ADAMTS13 activity at initial clinical remission

The ADAMTS13 activity was analyzed at initial clinical remission in only 32 out of the 76 patients studied. The ADAMTS13 activity showed 3 distinct courses: it either remained undetectable (<5%) in 13 patients (41%), became detectable but partially decreased (15 to 40%) in 12 patients (38%), or normal (50 to 100%) in 7 patients (21%). ADAMTS13 inhibitors in remission were detectable only in patients whose ADAMTS13 activity remained <5%, with titers either similar or decreased when compared to those of the acute episode (Fig.6).

When trying to correlate ADAMTS13 antibodies at presentation and ADAMTS13 activity at initial clinical remission; the presence of a high titer of ADAMTS13 inhibitor, either alone or combined with anti-ADAMTS13 antibodies of the IgG class at presentation, was associated with the persistence of an undetectable ADAMTS13 activity (<5%) in initial clinical remission (Fig.6).

## 4.4 Subclass distribution of IgG anti-ADAMTS13 antibodies

The biological function of IgG antibodies is determined by their specificity, affinity and subclasses. The IgG subclasses have different capacities to bind to cell surface Fcγ receptors (FcγRs) or to activate complement proteins, thus mediating different immunological effector functions[156]. Due to our findings that about 92% of the TTP patients have IgG anti-ADAMTS13 antibodies, we decided to characterize the IgG subclass distribution to elucidate a possible role of these antibodies in the pathomechanism leading to acquired TTP.

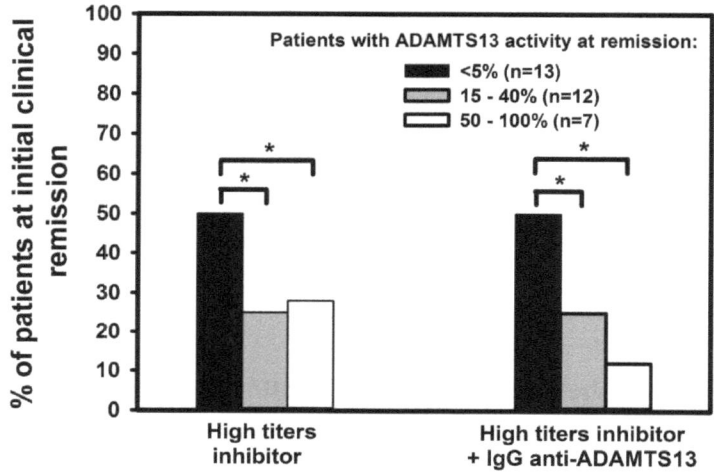

**Figure 6. Correlation between ADAMTS13 inhibitor titers at presentation and ADAMTS13 activity at initial clinical remission in patients with acquired TTP.**
Patients are grouped in 3 categories according to the level of ADAMTS13 activity at initial clinical remission: <5% (n = 13), between 15 and 40% (n = 12) and between 50 and 100% (n =7). At presentation, the presence of high titers of ADAMTS13 inhibitor, either alone or combined with IgG anti-ADAMTS13 antibodies, was more frequent in patients having undetectable ADAMTS13 activity (below 5%) at initial clinical remission when compared to patients having detectable ADAMTS13 activity. (*): significant statistical difference ($P < 0.05$) between both groups.

## 4.4.1 Subclass distribution of IgG anti-ADAMTS13 antibodies

The subclass distribution of anti-ADAMTS13 IgG antibodies was analyzed in the 58 patients who tested positive for anti-ADAMTS13 IgG antibodies in our in-house ELISA. From the 58 patients with acquired TTP tested, 44 patients were analyzed during the first episode and 14 during a relapse. IgG4 was detected in 90% of the patients (52/58, 90%), followed by IgG1 (30/58, 52%), IgG2 (29/58, 50%), and IgG3 (19/58, 33%).

When patients were subdivided by clinical outcome, 38/44 (86%) patients analyzed during the first event had IgG4 antibodies. IgG4 was found either alone (8/38, 21%) or with other IgG subclasses (30/38, 79%). Among the 30 patients in whom IgG4 was found with other IgG subclasses, the association with all four IgG subclasses (10/30, 33%) was the most prevalent finding, followed by association with IgG2 (7/30, 23%), IgG1 (5/30, 17%) and IgG3 (1/30, 3%). IgG4 was also found with IgG1 and IgG2 (4/30, 13%) and with IgG1 and IgG3 (3/30, 10%) (Fig. 7). No IgG4 was detected in 6/44 (14%) TTP patients who had predominantly IgG1 with IgG3 ($n = 2$), IgG2 ($n = 1$) or IgG2 and IgG3 ($n = 3$) (Fig. 7).

The IgG-subclass distribution in 14 patients analyzed during an acute relapsing event revealed IgG4 as the predominant IgG subclass (14/14, 100%); IgG4 was found either alone (9/14, 65%) or associated with IgG2 (3/14, 21%), IgG1 (1/14, 7%) or IgG1 and IgG2 (1/14, 7%), (Fig. 7).

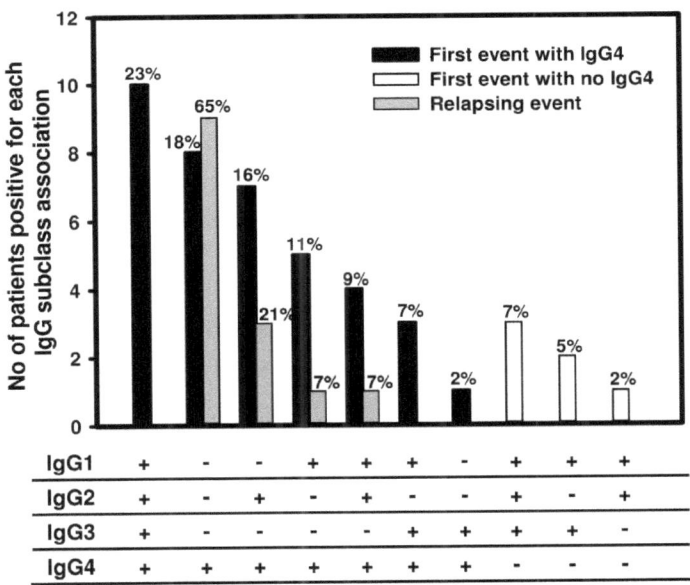

**Figure 7. Subclass distribution of anti-ADAMTS13 IgG antibodies in patients with acquired TTP.**

Fifty-eight patients with acute acquired TTP were analyzed for different IgG subclasses. The histograms show the frequencies of patients positive for each combination of IgG subclasses. Black and white bars represent patients analyzed during the first TTP episode ($n = 44$) with or without IgG4, respectively. Grey bars represent patients analyzed during a relapsing event ($n = 14$). Plus and minus signs denote the presence and absence of the subclass, respectively.

The IgG subclass distribution of 4/6 patients without detectable functional inhibitors showed IgG4 accompanied by IgG2 or IgG3 or IgG1 and IgG3, or all of them. The remaining two patients had no IgG4, with IgG1 being the most representative subclass.

To assess the contribution of any subclass to total IgG (IgG$_{sum}$), we calculated the relative concentration of each IgG subclass in a patient. Six of 58 patients were excluded from this calculation because their IgG4 OD values were outside the linear range. IgG4 was the most abundantly produced subclass, with levels ranging from 1% to 100% (Fig. 8A). IgG1 was the second most common subclass, with levels ranging from 11% to 92%, whereas, IgG2 and IgG3 formed only a small percentage of IgG$_{sum}$, with levels ranging from 4% to 26% and 1% to 30% for IgG2 and IgG3, respectively (Fig. 8A). In contrast to IgG4, IgG1 was never found as a single subclass; however, in the absence of IgG4, IgG1 constituted more than 85% of IgG$_{sum}$. The presence and abundance of IgG4 and IgG1 were inversely correlated ($r^2 = -0.927$, $P < 0.01$).

Because of the dominant presence of IgG4 antibodies in our patient population, IgE anti-ADAMTS13 antibodies were also assayed, as the production of IgG4 and IgE is induced by the same cytokines [interleukin (IL)-4 and IL-13], released by T-helper 2 cells[157]. None of the 17 patients with IgG4 as the only positive subclass had IgE antibodies against ADAMTS13, excluding a pathogenic role of IgE autoantibodies in TTP as described in, for example, bullous pemphigoid[158] or SLE[159].

## 4.4.2 Relation between the IgG subclass profile and the total anti-ADAMTS13 IgG antibody titers and ADAMTS13:Ag levels

When IgG$_{tot}$ was related to the IgG subclass profile, patients with IgG4 as the only subclass showed lower IgG$_{tot}$ titers (range 20-200) than patients with IgG4 combined with other IgG subclasses (Fig. 8B). The combination of IgG4 with one, two or more IgG subclasses was associated with the highest IgG$_{tot}$ titers (range 100-6400). This was even more pronounced in patients with undetectable IgG4 (range 1600-6400). Patients without detectable functional inhibitors generally had low IgG$_{tot}$ antibody titers (100-400), except for two patients who had undetectable IgG4 (1600 for both) (Fig. 8B).

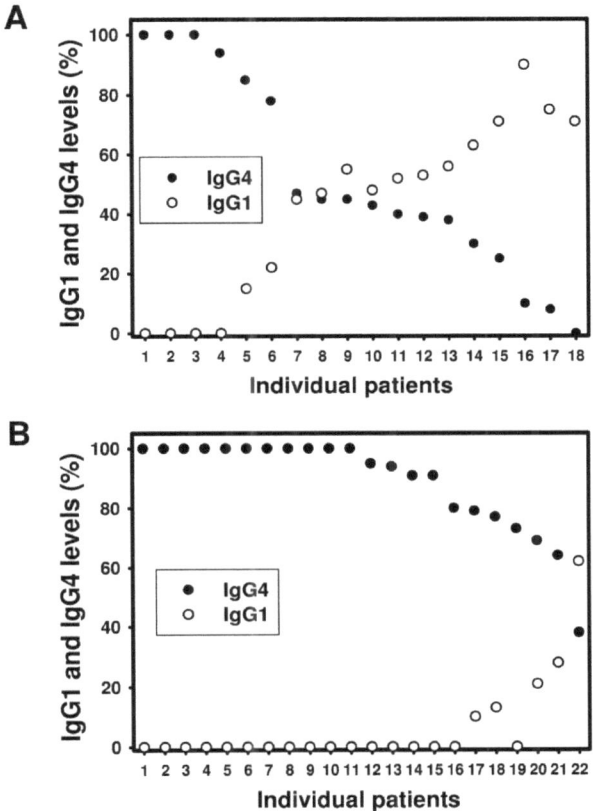

**Figure 8. Relative concentrations of anti-ADAMTS13 IgG subclasses and total IgG anti-ADAMTS13 antibody titers within a patient.**

(A) The relative concentration of the different IgG subclasses was calculated for plasma of 52 TTP patients. The individual IgG subclass distribution of each patient is shown. Patients are numbered 1-52 according to decreasing levels of IgG4. IgG4 and IgG1 are the dominating IgG subclasses. (B) Total IgG anti-ADAMTS13 antibody titers corresponding to each patient [numbered from 1 to 52 as in (A)]. In both (A) and (B), individual patient numbers are shown in steps of five.

The relationship between ADAMTS13:Ag levels and the IgG subclass profile was variable, with a trend towards lower ADAMTS13:Ag levels with increasing numbers of IgG subclasses. Patients with the lowest IgG4 levels (< 10%) or highest IgG1 levels (> 85%) had significantly lower ADAMTS13:Ag levels than patients with the highest IgG4 levels or IgG4 as the only subclass present ($P < 0.01$ and $P < 0.05$, respectively; the six patients with IgG4 OD values outside the linear range were excluded from this analysis).

### 4.4.3 Subclass distribution of anti-ADAMTS13 IgG antibodies and clinical outcome

We observed that 4 patients who had very low (< 5%) or undetectable IgG4 with high levels of IgG1 died during the first acute TTP event (Table 2). These patients also showed high anti-ADAMTS13 IgA antibodies titers, three of them in combination with anti-ADAMTS13 IgM antibodies.

This observation prompted us to search for an association between levels of IgG4 and IgG1 and recurrence of TTP. We analyzed 40 patients who were divided into three groups: those who had experienced only a single TTP episode [group 1; IgG4 and IgG1 median values were 44% (interquartile range (IQR) 30-85) and 50% (IQR 15-63), respectively], those who relapsed during 48 months of follow-up [group 2; IgG4 and IgG1 median values were 91% (IQR 72-95.5) and 0% (IQR 0-15), respectively] and those who had had relapse(s) before [group 3; IgG4 and IgG1 median values were 100% (IQR 91.2-100) and 0% (IQR 0-0), respectively] (Fig. 9) (for inclusion criteria, see Methodology, chapter 3.9). High levels of IgG4 were associated with relapse ($P = 0.03$ and $P = 0.001$ for comparison between groups 1 and 2 and groups 1 and 3, respectively).

Likewise, patients with undetectable or very low IgG1 levels experienced more TTP events than patients with detectable (moderate or low) levels ($P = 0.005$ and $P < 0.001$ for comparison between groups 1 and 2 and groups 1 and 3, respectively).

Taken together, our findings suggest that patients with high levels of IgG4 and undetectable IgG1 are more prone to relapse than patients with low levels of IgG4 and detectable IgG1.

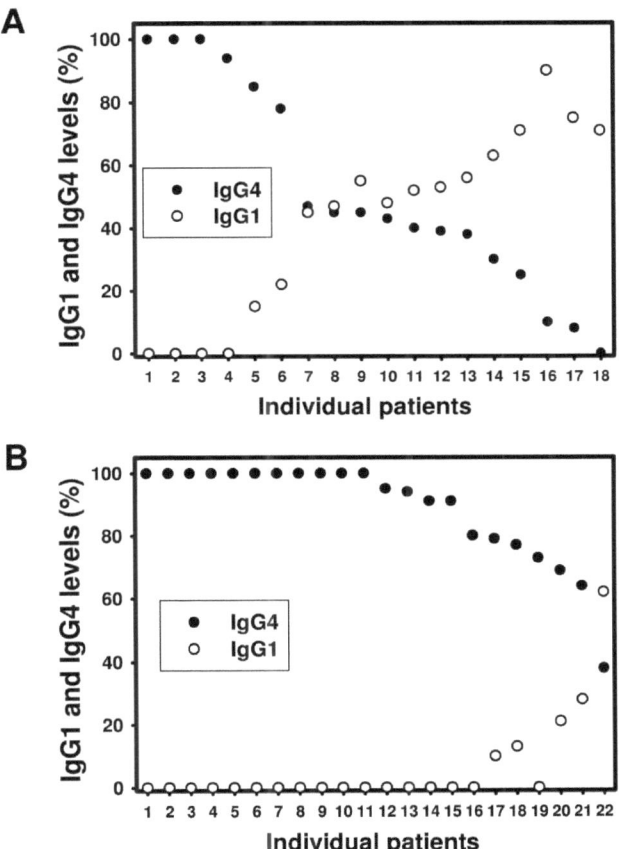

**Figure 9. Levels of IgG1 and IgG4 anti-ADAMTS13 antibodies in patients with acute acquired TTP.**

(A) Patients who had experienced only a single TTP event. (B) Patients who relapsed during the 48 months of follow-up or had had relapse(s) including patients without further relapses during follow-up and patients lost to follow-up after the acute relapsing event.

Table 2. ADAMTS13 laboratory findings and clinical outcome in patients with very low (<5%) or undetectable levels of IgG4 and high levels of IgG1

| Patient N°* | ADAMTS13:Ac (U/mL) | ADAMTS13 inhibitor | ADAMTS13:Ag (ng/mL) | IgG anti-ADAMTS13 (titer) | IgM anti-ADAMTS13 (titer) | IgA anti-ADAMTS13 (titer) | IgG1 (%) | IgG4 (%) | Outcome |
|---|---|---|---|---|---|---|---|---|---|
| 49 | <0.05 | High | <65 | 6400 | 3200 | 12800 | 92 | 0 | Death |
| 50 | <0.05 | Low | <65 | 3200 | 0 | 0 | 92 | 0 | Remission |
| 48 | <0.05 | Neg. | <65 | 1600 | 0 | 51200 | 91 | 0 | Death |
| 52 | <0.05 | Neg. | <65 | 1600 | 50 | 800 | 85 | 0 | Death |
| 46 | <0.05 | Low | <65 | 3200 | 0 | 3200 | 88 | 1 | Remission |
| 45 | <0.05 | Low | 83 | 1600 | 20 | 3200 | 78 | 3 | Death |
| 47 | <0.05 | Low | 560 | 200 | 0 | 0 | 71 | 0 | Remission |

ADAMTS13:Ac, ADAMTS13 activity; ADAMTS13:Ag, ADAMTS13 antigen; Neg., Negative. *Patient' numbers correspond to the individual numbers in Fig. 4. All patients had idiopathic thrombotic thrombocytopenic purpura

## 4.5 Detection of circulating ADAMTS13-anti-ADAMTS13 antibody immune complexes in patients with acquired TTP

During the establishment of our in-house ELISA to quantify ADAMTS13 antigen levels[51], we observed that removal from plasma of anti-ADAMTS13 IgG antibodies by Protein G also completely removed any measurable residual ADAMTS13 antigen, indicating that all ADAMTS13 was bound to IgG antibodies. These findings were the first evidence for the presence of soluble ADAMTS13-specific immune complexes (ICs) in plasma from patients with acquired TTP.

These observations prompted us to establish two types of assays to experimentally detect circulating ADAMTS13-specific ICs: one based on co-immunoprecipitation of ADAMTS13 with IgG antibodies using Protein G and the second one based on ELISA methodology.

## 4.5.1 Detection of circulating ADAMTS13-anti-ADAMTS13 antibody immune complexes by co-immunoprecipitation

For co-immunoprecipitation (Co-IP) experiments, plasma samples from all those patients with acute acquired TTP ($n$=16) were included where sufficient amounts of plasma were still available. As negative controls, plasmas from healthy individuals, different batches of pooled NHP and human serum albumin (HSA, 50 µg/mL) spiked with recombinant ADAMTS13 (rADAMTS13, 2 µg/mL) were also analyzed.

All samples were subjected to immunoprecipitation with Protein G and co-isolated ADAMTS13 was detected by Western blot analysis using an affinity-purified polyclonal rabbit anti-human ADAMTS13 antibody. The sensitivity of this antibody to detect rADAMTS13 in a blot is approximately 0.5 ng.

ADAMTS13 was not detectable in the protein G-bound total IgG derived from healthy individual plasmas, pooled NHP or HSA spiked with rADAMTS13 (Fig. 10A). ADAMTS13 was however detectable in most of the 16 TTP-derived samples (Fig. 10B) suggesting the specific detection of circulating ADAMTS13-IgG ICs.

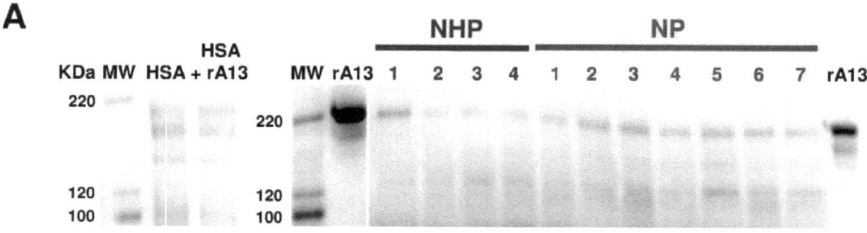

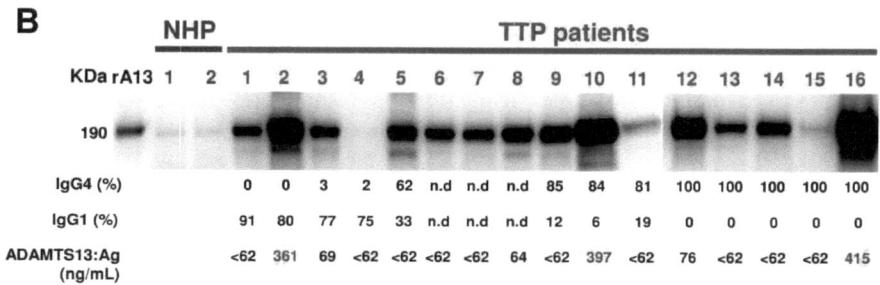

**Figure 10. Detection of circulating ADAMTS13-anti-ADAMTS13 antibody immune complexes (ICs) in TTP patients by co-immunoprecipitation.**

Circulating ADAMTS13-specific ICs were analyzed by co-immunoprecipitation of ADAMTS13 with Protein G-bound IgG followed by Western blot analysis to detect ADAMTS13. The position of ADAMTS13 in the gels was determined by loading 1 ng of recombinant ADAMTS13 (rA13). (A) Healthy individuals (NP), different batches of pooled normal human plasma (NHP), human serum albumin (HSA; 50 µg/mL) and HSA spiked with 2 µg/mL of recombinant ADAMTS13 (HSA + rA13). (B) TTP patients. Two batches of NHP served as negative control. The relative percentage of IgG1 and IgG4 antibodies and ADAMTS13:Ag values of the samples are also shown. Each lane contains equal amounts of total IgG.

Except for one patient (Fig. 10B; TTP 4), circulating ADAMTS13-IgG ICs were detected in all plasma samples ($n$=9) where free ADAMTS13:Ag levels were not detectable (Fig. 10B). An interesting observation is that 3 patients who had measurable residual ADAMTS13:Ag levels (levels between 361 – 415 ng/mL) showed also higher IC levels compared to those patients with no detectable protein (Fig. 10B; TTP 2, TTP 10 and TTP 16), suggesting that the ELISA employed to quantify ADAMTS13:Ag levels is also detecting circulating ADAMTS13-specific ICs at least to some extent, in line with a previous report[51].

No differences could be observed when the presence and relative amounts of circulating ADAMTS13-IgG ICs were compared with those of the subclasses of the free anti-ADAMTS13 IgG antibodies. Patients having mainly IgG1 antibodies (Fig. 10B; TTP 1 to 5) had similar amount of ICs as patients having mainly IgG4 antibodies (Fig. 10B; TTP 9 to 16). These observations may suggest that the formation and clearance of ADAMTS13-IgG ICs is independent of the IgG subclass involved in IC formation.

Patients with low levels of free IgG anti-ADAMTS13 antibodies (detectable only with a commercial ELISA kit) also contained ADAMTS13-IgG ICs (Fig. 10B; TTP 6 to 8).

## 4.5.2 Detection of circulating ADAMTS13-anti-ADAMTS13 antibody immune complexes by ELISA

The positive findings obtained with the Co-IP experiments and considering our previous observation that an ADAMTS13:Ag ELISA was able to indirectly detect ADAMTS13-specific ICs, we aimed to establish an ELISA-based assay that should detect and characterize the immunoglobulin fraction of the circulating ADAMTS13-specific ICs.

For this, the basic set-up of the in-house ELISA to quantify ADAMTS13:Ag levels was modified at the detection step to visualize the antibody fraction of the immune complex. Briefly, a polyclonal rabbit anti-ADAMTS13 antibody is used to capture any ADAMTS13-anti-ADAMTS13 antibody ICs present in the plasma and the immunoglobulin fraction of the IC is detected by means of enzymatically-labeled anti-human IgG1-4 or IgA antibodies. The major limitation of this ELISA is that only ICs bearing an ADAMTS13 with free available epitopes will be detected.

The presence of circulating ADAMTS13-specific ICs was analyzed in 60 healthy donor plasmas to establish assay cut-off values. Circulating ADAMTS13-specific ICs were also tested in a total of 57 out of 76 TTP patients for which plasma samples were available. The levels of ADAMTS13-specific ICs were expressed as ratio between the OD values obtained with the tested plasma and OD values of a pooled NHP.

Circulating IgG- and IgA-ADAMTS13 ICs were detected in 47/57 (82%) and 13/53 (25%) of the TTP patients, respectively. When the IgG subclass distribution of ADAMTS13-IgG-specific ICs were analyzed; 41/47 (87%) of the TTP patients showed an IgG4-IC, 19/47 (40%) an IgG2-IC, 15/47 (32%) an IgG1-IC and only 7/47 (15%) of the patients an IgG3-IC (Fig. 11). Comparing the levels of ADAMTS13-specific ICs between TTP patients and healthy donors revealed a statistically significant difference for IgG1, IgG2, IgG4 and IgA ICs ($P < 0.001$ for IgG1, IgG2, IgG4 and IgA, respectively), but not for IgG3 ($P = 0.456$).

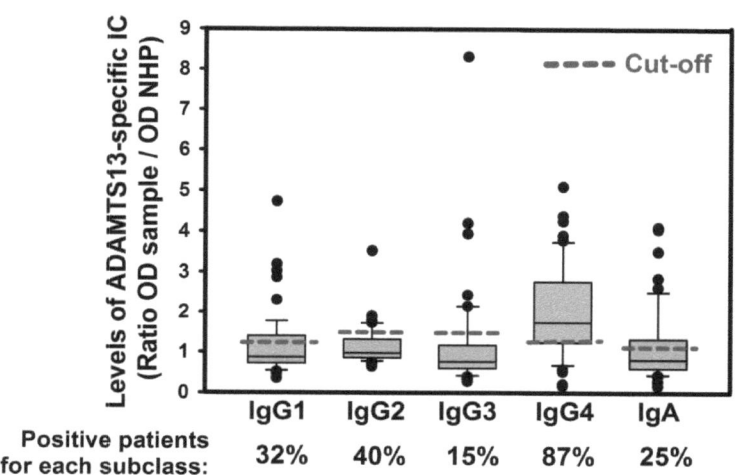

**Figure 11. Detection of circulating ADAMTS13-anti-ADAMTS13 antibody ICs in patients with acute acquired TTP by ELISA.**

Box plot of the distribution of circulating IgG1 to IgG4- and IgA-ADAMTS13 specific ICs in plasma from 57 TTP patients. The IC levels are presented as ratio between the OD of the sample and the OD of a pooled NHP (dilution 1 to 20). The dashed lines represent the normal cut-off value for each ELISA. The bottom, median and top lines of the box mark the $25^{th}$, $50^{th}$, and $75^{th}$ percentiles, respectively. The vertical line shows the range of values comprised between the $5^{th}$ and $95^{th}$ percentiles and the dots represent outlier values. The percentage of positive TTP patients for each subclass of ADAMTS13-specific IC is shown at the bottom.

In 68% of the patients tested positive for IgG-ICs a correlation between the subclasses of the free IgG anti-ADAMTS13 antibodies found in the plasma and the subclasses of the IgG-containing ICs was observed. Importantly, all patients that were tested negative for free IgG4 antibodies also tested negative for IgG4-containing ICs. In 8/12 (67%) of the TTP patients tested positive for free IgA anti-ADAMTS13 antibodies also tested positive for IgA-containing ICs.

Interestingly, in 2 out of 6 and 5 out of 41 patients tested negative for IgG and IgA anti-ADAMTS13 antibodies, respectively, circulating ADAMTS13-specific ICs (involving IgG2, IgG4 or IgA) were detected by ELISA. This indicated that a negative finding of free anti-ADAMTS13 antibodies in plasma may be due to the sequestration of these antibodies in ICs.

In only 6 patients circulating ADAMTS13-IgG-specific ICs were not detected although free IgG anti-ADAMTS13 antibodies and practically no ADAMTS13:Ag were present.

Eight out of 9 patients who tested positive for free IgG anti-ADAMTS13 antibodies only by the commercial ELISA were tested positive for IgG4-IC suggesting that our in-house ELISA is not detecting low levels of free IgG4 antibodies. These observations confirm previous findings that the goat anti-human IgG antibody used to visualize IgG in the in-house ELISA detected IgG4 with ~50% lower sensitivity than IgG1-3 antibodies.

Four patients tested negative for anti-ADAMTS13 antibodies also tested negative for all classes and subclasses of ICs (IgG1-4 and IgA).

## 4.5.3 Detection of complement fixing immune complexes by binding to immobilized C1q

The complement subcomponent C1q binds to the Fc region of complexed IgG or IgM thereby triggering the activation of the classical complement pathway. Based on these properties, we used a commercially available C1q binding ELISA to evaluate if ADAMTS13-containing ICs are able to activate complement. Plasmas derived from 37 TTP patients included in the current study and from 3 healthy individuals were tested. In 6 out of 37 (16%) patients circulating ICs bound to immobilized C1q were detected (Fig. 12). Borderline and negative values were obtained for 6/37 (16%) and 25/37 (68%) of the patients, respectively (Fig. 12). All 3 healthy individuals tested also negative. Since C1q is efficient in binding ICs only when containing IgG subclasses 1 to 3, the results are in accordance with the observed high prevalence (87%) of circulating ADAMS13-IgG4-specific ICs.

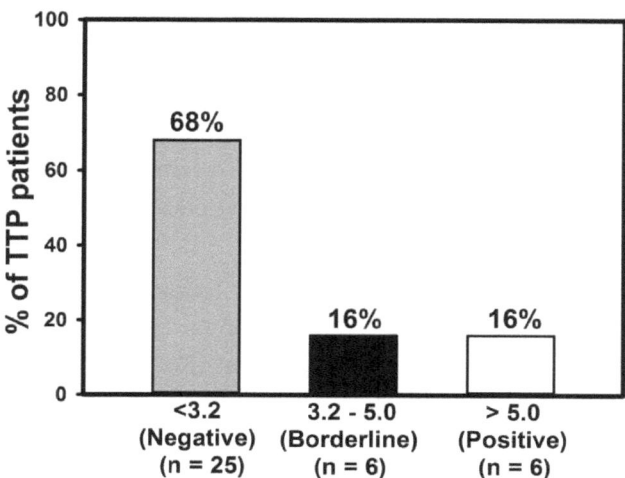

**Figure 12. Detection of complement fixing ICs by binding to immobilized C1q**
The levels of circulating ICs (µg EQ/mL) binding to immobilized C1q was evaluated in 37 TTP plasma samples by ELISA. The negative cut-off value of the assay was 3.2 µg Eq/mL, samples with 3.2-5.0 µg Eq/mL were judged as borderline and samples with values above 5.0 µg Eq/mL were judged as positive.

## 4.6 Binding of human IgG4 to rabbit anti-ADAMTS13 antibody

During the establishment of the ELISA to detect circulating ADAMS13-IgG4-specific ICs, undesired high background signals were reached when testing either pooled NHP or individual healthy donor plasmas. These findings might have been caused by the potential presence of naturally occurring circulating ADAMS13-IgG4-specific ICs in the healthy population or by a propensity of human IgG4 present in normal plasma to bind rabbit IgG antibodies.

The first possibility was explored comparing pooled NHP with an ADAMTS13-depleted pooled NHP (depleted-NHP) prepared as previously described[51], and the second by using a commercially available purified human IgG4 (hIgG4) preparation in a concentration range comparable to the final amount of IgG4 present at each tested dilution of pooled NHP. Interestingly, similar results were obtained with both set-ups (Fig. 13), indicating that hIgG4 is able to bind to coated rabbit IgG in a dose-dependent manner, thereby causing the high background signals in the ELISA.

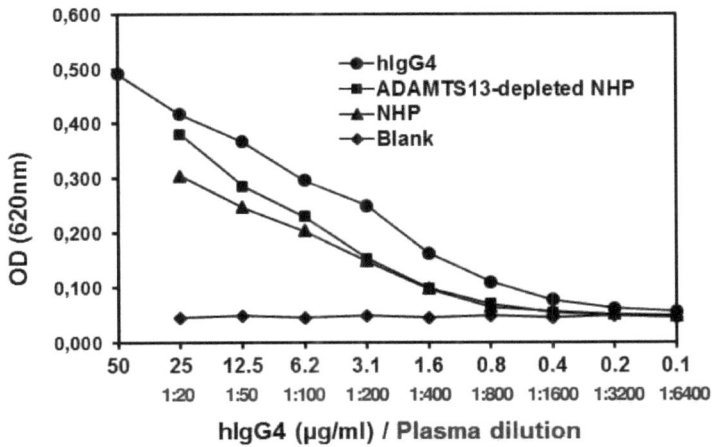

**Figure 13. Binding of human IgG4 to coated rabbit IgG antibodies.**

Serial dilutions of pooled NHP and ADAMTS13-depleted NHP (indicated in blue color) as well as purified human IgG4 (hIgG4) at concentrations comparable to the final amount of IgG4 present at each tested dilution of pooled NHP (indicated in black color) were allowed to bind to coated rabbit IgG. As negative control (blank), blocking buffer was used as a sample.

Similar results were obtained when rabbit IgG antibodies in solution were allowed to bind to coated hIgG4. Moreover, hIgG4 in solution was capable of competing with rADAMTS13 for binding to coated rabbit anti-ADAMTS13 IgG (data not shown).

This conclusion was further corroborated by pre-incubating pooled NHP, ADAMTS13-depleted-NHP and hIgG4 with a monoclonal anti-human IgG4 (Fc-specific) antibody in a final concentration of 11 μg/mL. The binding of IgG4 to coated rabbit IgG was equally inhibited in all three samples but not in control samples pre-incubated with BSA (differences approximately 5-fold; data not shown). These preliminary results suggested that hIgG4 is able to bind to coated rabbit IgG via its Fc fragment because the Fc-specific anti-human IgG4 antibody was able to abrogate the binding.

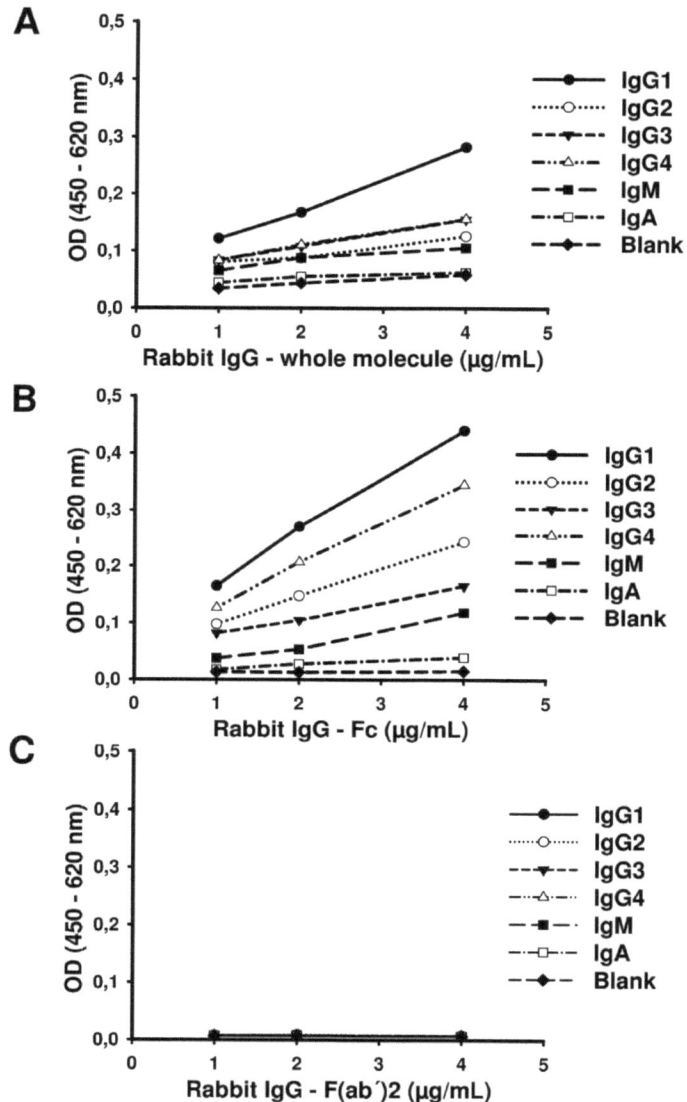

**Figure 14. Binding of rabbit IgG antibodies to coated human immunoglobulins.**

Horseradish peroxidase (HRP)-labeled whole rabbit IgG, IgG (Fab')2 or IgG Fc antibodies were allowed to bind to coated purified human IgG1-4, IgM or IgA antibodies. (A) Binding of whole rabbit IgG to Igs. (B) Binding of rabbit IgG Fc to Igs. (C) Binding of rabbit IgG (Fab')2 to Igs.

We next explored the nature of the hIgG4-rabbit IgG interaction and also the potential binding of other human immunoglobulins (IgM, IgA or IgG1-3) to rabbit IgG. For this, HRP-labeled whole rabbit IgG, HRP-labelled IgG (Fab')2 fragment and HRP-labelled IgG Fc fragment were allowed to bind to coated purified human IgG1-4, IgM or IgA antibodies. The results confirmed that the binding of rabbit IgG antibodies to human IgG4 is mediated via its Fc rather than its F(ab')2 portion (Fig. 14). Interestingly, we also observed an increased dose-dependent binding of rabbit IgG (Fc fragment) to coated human IgG1 and to a lesser extent to IgG2, IgG3 and IgM. No binding was observed to IgA (Fig. 14).

Because of these findings, we assayed for binding of human IgG1-3 to rabbit IgG antibodies. Different concentration of human IgG1-3 (comparable to those of each tested dilution of pooled NHP) and diluted pooled NHP were allowed to bind to coated rabbit IgG antibodies. Neither IgG1, IgG2 nor IgG3 had the ability to bind to rabbit IgG under the conditions used (data not shown).

## 4.7 Detection of anti-ADAMTS13 antibodies and circulating ADAMTS13-immune complexes in a follow-up of a patient with refractory TTP

The dynamic course of anti-ADAMTS13 antibodies and circulating ADAMTS13-IC during treatment was investigated in a patient suffering from refractory TTP[130]. Throughout the follow-up until the decease of the patient at day 64, plasma samples were collected daily before treatment and ADAMTS13-related parameters were determined. ADAMTS13:Ac and ADAMTS13:Ag were undetectable at most time points. High inhibitor titers were measured during the first two weeks and declined to low levels thereafter. Anti-ADAMTS13 antibodies of the IgG, IgM and IgA class were detected concomitantly (Fig. 15). For IgG and IgA antibodies, high to moderate titers were found practically throughout the entire observation time.

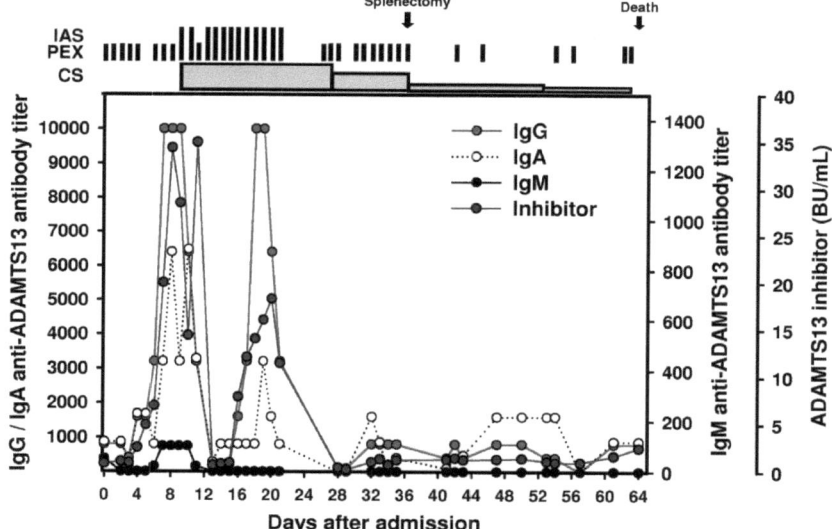

**Figure 15. Dynamic course of anti-ADAMTS13 antibodies in a patient with refractory TTP.**
Dynamic course of anti-ADAMTS13 antibody titers (IgG, IgM, IgA and functional inhibitor (BU/mL)) during the two months follow-up. The treatment regimen including plasma exchange (PEX), immunoadsorption (IAS), corticosteroids (CS), and splenectomy is shown above the diagram.

By contrast, IgM antibodies were detected only at the beginning and with low titers. The anti-ADAMTS13 IgG subclass profile showed prevalence of IgG1 (82%) and very low levels of IgG2 (7%) and IgG3 (11%) antibodies, while IgG4 was undetectable. This antibody profile did not change during the course of the disease.

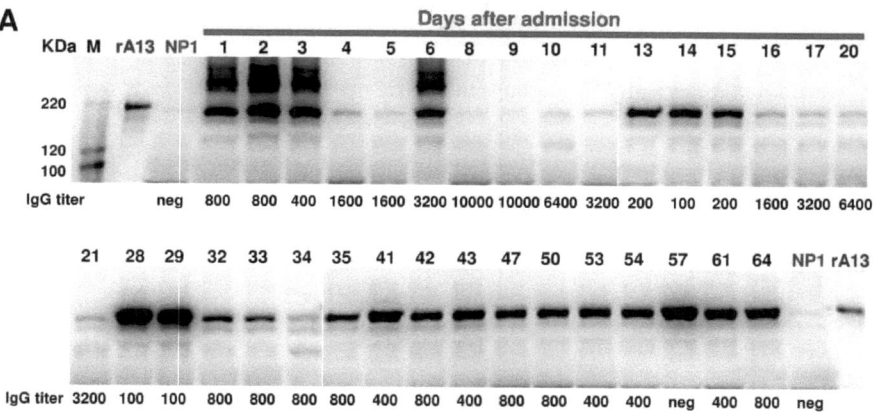

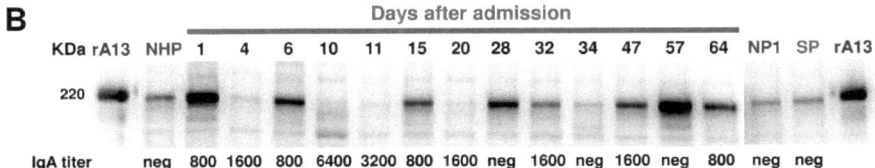

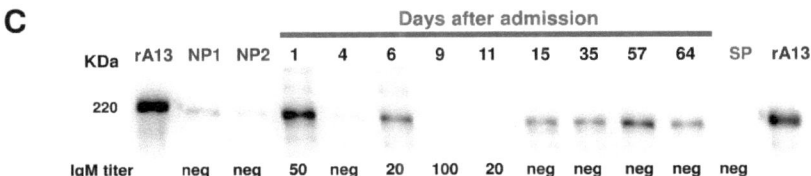

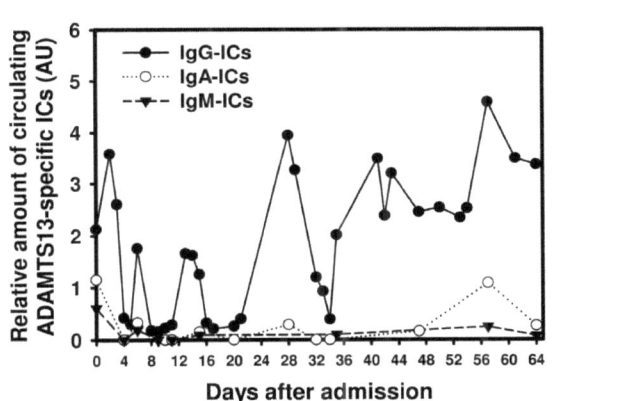

**Figure 16. Dynamic course of circulating ADAMTS13-specific ICs in a patient with refractory TTP.**

Immunoblots showing the course of circulating (A) ADAMTS13-IgG ICs, (B) ADAMTS13-IgA ICs and (C) ADAMTS13-IgM ICs. Recombinant ADAMTS13 (rA13, 1ng/well) was used as negative control. Pooled NHP (NHP), a single healthy donors (NP) and human serum albumin (HSA; 50 µg/mL) spiked with 2 µg/mL of rA13 (SP) were used as negative controls. M denotes the molecular weight marker. Each lane contains equal amounts of total IgG. The corresponding anti-ADAMTS13 antibody titers are also shown in the lower panel of each blot. (D) Relative amount of circulating ADAMTS13-specific ICs after densitometric quantification using rA13 (1 ng) as standard. AU denotes arbitrary units.

The presence of ADAMTS13-specific IgG, IgM and IgA ICs was investigated by Co-IP and ELISA. The former method detected ADAMTS13-specific ICs for all the 3 classes of antibodies. By determining the relative amounts of circulating ICs through scanning of the luminograms (Fig. 16A-D), it appeared that the plasma concentration of the IgG-ICs is higher than that of the IgM- and IgA-ICs. Interestingly, ADAMTS13-specific ICs followed an inverse kinetics to that of the measured free antibody titers. ICs were detectable most of the time but became apparently undetectable when the titers of the free antibodies rose (Fig. 16A-D). Notably, low amounts of IgM-ICs were detected at most time points although no free IgM antibodies were detected after day 12 (Fig. 16A-D).

The presence of ICs was also analyzed by ELISA in the sample collected at day 1. Circulating IgG1-ICs, IgG3-ICs and IgA-ICs were detected. IgM-ICs were not investigated by ELISA. A correlation could again be observed when the classes and subclasses of free ADAMTS13 antibodies were compared with those of the immunoglobulin forming the ICs.

## 4.8 Detection of anti-CD36 antibodies in TTP patients

Previous studies have shown that approximately 70% of the TTP patients have autoantibodies against the membrane antigen CD36[148-150;153]. In these studies, platelet lysates were used as source of human CD36 and the presence of anti-CD36 antibodies was evaluated by either Western blot with patient's plasma as first antibody or by immunoprecipitation of patient's plasma antibodies with platelet lysates-derived CD36. Alternatively, a Dot blot using purified platelet-derived CD36 as protein source was performed.

The published high incidence of anti-CD36 antibodies in TTP patients prompted us to develop a more sensitive assay based on ELISA technique to detect these antibodies in the plasma from TTP patients. The source of human CD36 used to coat the ELISA plates was a commercially available full-length recombinant human CD36 (rCD36) expressed in human embryonic kidney cells (HEK 293).

The presence of anti-CD36 antibodies was investigated in 57 of the 76 TTP patients included in the current study and in 36 additional TTP patients whose plasma samples became available at a later point in time.

A total of 63 healthy donor samples were analyzed to establish assay cut-off values. In the absence of any human-derived positive control, a monoclonal rat anti-human CD36 antibody directed against the extracellular part of human CD36 was used as positive control to allow following the assay performance.

Circulating anti-CD36 antibodies were detected in only 7/93 (8%) of the TTP patients and in 2/63 (3%) of the healthy donors (Fig.17). From the 57 patients included in the study described in previous chapters, only 3 patients tested positive. There was no statistically significant difference ($P < 0.197$) between healthy donors and TTP patients when the levels of anti-CD36 antibodies (expressed as ratio between OD of the tested sample and the OD of a pooled NHP) were compared (Fig.17).

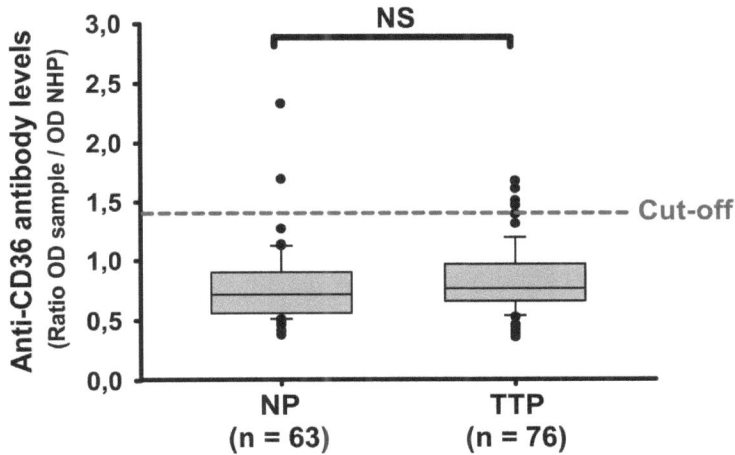

**Figure 17. Detection of anti-CD36 antibodies in patients with acquired TTP.**
Box plot of the distribution of anti-CD36 antibodies in plasma from 63 healthy donors (NP) and 93 patients with acquired TTP. The anti-CD36 antibodies levels are presented as ratio between the OD of the sample and the OD of a pooled NHP. The dashed line represents the normal ELISA cut-off value. The bottom, median and top lines of the box mark the $25^{th}$, $50^{th}$, and $75^{th}$ percentiles, respectively. The vertical line shows the range of values comprised between the $5^{th}$ and $95^{th}$ percentiles and the dots represent outlier values. NS= non-significant statistical difference between both groups.

For 3 out of the 7 TTP plasma samples tested positive for anti-CD36 antibodies competitive inhibition experiments between immobilized rCD36 and rCD36 in solution could be performed. Specificity of the detected anti-CD36 antibody could be shown in 2 samples, whereas the third sample displayed inhibition also with different protein sources used as negative control (rADAMTS13 and BSA).

In summary, we confirmed the detection of anti-CD36 antibodies in 2 out 3 TTP patients by our in-house ELISA but not with the commercial kit. The positivity of 4 TTP patients could not be confirmed with any additional assay due to unavailability of plasma sample.

# 5- DISCUSSION

The pathogenesis of acquired idiopathic TTP is characterized by severe ADAMTS13 deficiency due to the presence of circulating autoantibodies directed against ADAMTS13 that may or may not inhibit its functional activity[130-132]. The main goal of the present study was to characterize the immune response against ADAMTS13 in a well-defined cohort of 76 adult TTP patients who underwent a first acute episode (n=57) or who had an acute relapsing event (n=19).

## *Characterization of the free anti-ADAMTS13 antibodies*

Anti-ADAMTS13 antibodies were identified in 71 out of the 76 (93%) TTP patients. IgG, IgM and IgA antibodies were detected in 92%, 7% and 17% of the patients, respectively (Fig. 5). The IgG and IgM findings are in agreement with a previous study of our group in which IgG and IgM antibodies were detected in 97% and 11% of the TTP patients, respectively[132]. Subsequent studies reported a similar prevalence of IgG[120;131;133;136] and IgM[136] antibodies in TTP patients.

This is the first study on IgA antibodies against ADAMTS13 in TTP patients. The frequency rate of 17% for IgA antibodies found here[160] is very similar to the 19% of a more recent study conducted by Pos *et al*[136]. Interestingly, one patient from our cohort with a positive functional inhibitor had detectable antibodies only of the IgA class, suggesting that IgA antibodies can also have inhibiting activity against ADAMTS13. High levels of IgA antibodies were recently found to be associated with mortality[161]. In line with this observation, we observed that high levels of IgA antibodies were present in 3 out of 4 death cases. Pathogenic IgA autoantibodies are described in patients suffering of SLE and antiphospholipid syndrome and they are considered a risk factor for development of thrombosis[162;163]. The clinical significance and pathogenic potential of IgA antibodies in acquired TTP is however unknown and further studies are needed to assess their contribution to the pathogenesis of TTP.

Inhibitory antibodies were found in 92% of the patients while the rate of non-inhibitory antibodies in this study was only 8%. These data indicate that a majority of the anti-ADAMTS13 antibodies is inhibitory in vitro and, since most of them target domains that are required for ADAMTS13 proteolytic activity[134;137], these antibodies are probably also inhibitory in vivo. On the other hand, the detection of non-inhibitory antibodies in samples from patients with acquired TTP may be assay dependent and their frequency of occurrence remains controversial. Depending on the study, the prevalence of non-inhibitory antibodies lies between 7% and 29%[120;131;133]. Since most of the functional assays used for functional inhibitor detection suffer from a lack of sensitivity, antibodies with a low affinity and/or concentration may be missed, thereby overestimating the rate of acquired TTP patients with non-inhibitory antibodies.

Another novel finding of this study was the characterization of the subclasses of anti-ADAMTS13 IgG antibodies. The IgG subclass distribution of anti-ADAMTS13 IgG antibodies was investigated in 58 out of 76 TTP patients included in this cohort. In a remarkable number of patients (17/58), IgG4 was the only subtype that could be detected, implying that IgG4 plays a dominant role in the pathogenesis of autoimmune TTP. The second most frequent subtype was IgG1, while IgG2 and IgG3 were less represented (Fig. 7). A similar prevalence of IgG subclasses in a cohort of 48 acquired TTP patients was recently reported[136]. Importantly, IgG4 antibodies were found in all relapsed patients suggesting a chronic stimulation of the immune system since IgG4 is mainly produced under conditions of chronic antigen exposure driven by a T-helper 2 immune response[164]. There was also an inverse correlation between the frequency and abundance of IgG4 and IgG1 antibodies ($P < 0.01$) and we consider this inverse relation to be an important factor in the pathophysiology of acquired TTP due to the distinct biological functions exerted by these two subclasses. IgG1 is known to bind to both complement C1q and FcγRs thus leading to activation of the classical complement pathway and immune and endothelial cells, whereas IgG4 has poor ability to induce both complement and cell activation[156].

The ELISAs used in this thesis to detect anti-ADAMTS13 antibodies were developed in-house and utilized immobilized recombinant ADAMTS13 to bind the various antibodies. Compared to the method published previously by our group for the detection of anti-ADAMTS13 IgG and IgM antibodies[132], we have introduced a slight modification to the basic set-up so as to allow the additional detection of the different IgG subclasses, IgA and IgE anti-ADAMTS13 antibodies. The method was able to detect both inhibitory and non-inhibitory autoantibodies. Thus, it appears suitable for treatment monitoring because it is easy to perform, the results can be available within a few hours, and seems to have a much greater sensitivity than the classical inhibitor assay due to the detection also of non-inhibitory antibodies. In the future, the sensitivity of the ELISA could be further improved by replacing the alkaline-phosphatase-conjugated secondary antibodies by a horseradish peroxidase-conjugated one.

Taken together, our findings indicate that the autoimmune response against ADAMTS13 is polyclonal and heterogeneous with different classes and subclasses of autoantibodies playing key roles in the patho-mechanism of acquired TTP. Clearly, further studies are needed to investigate the specific pathogenic role of each antibody type.

## *Anti-CD36 antibody incidence is not correlated with acquired TTP*

Based on reports on a high incidence of anti-CD36 antibodies in acquired TTP patients[148-150], we developed an ELISA assay to analyze our own cohort for presence of these autoantibodies. Anti-CD36 antibodies were found in only 8% of the TTP patients analyzed and in 3% of the healthy donor control group. This result was in contrast to the frequency of about 70% observed previously by other authors[148-150].

This gross discrepancy in the frequency of detected anti-CD36 antibodies is likely due to differences in the methods employed for antibody detection. We performed an ELISA using recombinant CD36 as protein source and the biotin-streptavidin system for detection, which is well-known to confer a high sensitivity to the ELISA detection. In the past, Western blot analysis was employed, with platelet extracts as source for CD36 and patient's plasma as a first antibody. This may well lead to a high incidence of false positives due to binding of antibodies to unrelated proteins. Furthermore, we have tested a total of 93 TTP plasma samples whereas in previous studies a range between 10 to 35 patients had been used[148-150;153]. Such differences in population number could also introduce a bias in the observed high frequency of positive samples. We are therefore confident that our data show that acquired TTP patients do not exhibit an increased incidence of anti-CD36 antibodies.

## *Presence of ADAMTS13-specific circulating ICs in acquired TTP patients*

Elevated levels of soluble circulating autoantibody-antigen immune complexes are a hallmark of certain autoimmune diseases such as SLE, rheumathoid arthritis, antiphospholipid syndrome, vasculitis, and glomerulonephritis[165]. Also acquired TTP has been thought to be an IC-mediated disease ever since the isolation of ADAMTS13-inhibiting IgG antibodies from plasma of TTP patients[35]. Early reports attributed the benefit of PEX therapy in TTP patients to the removal of potential circulating ICs[166;167] but the presence of circulating ICs in TTP patients remained controversial[168;169].

A previous study by our group showed that removal of anti-ADAMTS13 IgG antibodies from plasma of TTP patients also removed any measurable residual ADAMTS13 antigen suggesting for the first time that the ELISA employed to quantify ADAMTS13 antigen levels is also detecting, at least to some extent, ADAMTS13-specific ICs[51]. Similar observations were recently reported by Yang *et al*[170] using a commercially available kit to quantify ADAMTS13 antigen levels. Based on these observations, we decided to investigate the presence of circulating ADAMTS13-specific ICs in more detail using two different approaches: one based on co-immunoprecipitation of ADAMTS13 with IgG antibodies using Protein G and the second one based on ELISA methodology.

Co-immunoprecipitation experiments showed the presence of circulating ADAMTS13-IgG ICs in plasma of patients with TTP but not in healthy donors (Fig. 10). IgG-ICs were detected in patients with or without detectable free ADAMTS13 antigen, indicating that the absence of measurable ADAMTS13 antigen might be due to sequestration in ICs. These findings also suggest that our in-house ADAMTS13 antigen ELISA is detecting ICs only in those patients whose complexed ADAMTS13 still conserves available epitopes for binding to both the capture and detection anti-ADAMTS13 antibodies. The availability of free epitopes might indicate the presence of small-sized ICs. Moreover, IgG-ICs were detected in patients having either IgG4 or IgG1 anti-ADAMTS13 antibodies as predominant IgG subclasses, suggesting an apparently equal avidity of some IgG subclasses of antibodies for ADAMTS13. These experiments confirmed our previous findings and suggested that formation of circulating ADAMTS13-IgG-specific ICs is a common feature of acquired TTP.

We found IgG4 as the predominant subclass of free autoantibodies in TTP patients. Since this IgG subclass is the least effective in terms of final effector functions under normal conditions, we reasoned that the lack of detection of other free IgG subclasses might be due to their sequestration in ICs. Such circulating ICs (containing IgG1-3 or IgA antibodies) would also better explain the pathogenesis of TTP than the exclusive presence of rather harmless IgG4 antibodies. For their detection, we developed ELISA-based assays where a polyclonal anti-ADAMTS13 antibody was used to capture the ICs through ADAMTS13 and the immunoglobulin constituents (IgG1-4 and IgA) of the ICs were detected by enzyme-labeled antibodies specific for the Ig classes and subclasses. The ELISA set-up used was clearly suitable and sufficiently sensitive for the detection of ICs. A limitation of this ELISA setup is however its underestimation of the real concentration of circulating ICs in case of large-sized ICs harboring more than one ADAMTS13 molecule and ICs with no free ADAMTS13 epitopes available.

Characterization of circulating ICs by ELISA revealed the presence of IgG- and IgA-containing ICs in 81% and 23% of the 57 patients with TTP investigated, respectively. Moreover, in the patients tested positive for IgG-ICs, a substantial overlap between free and IC-sequestered IgG subclasses was observed. IgG4-ICs were most frequent (72%), followed by IgG2-ICs (37%) and IgG1-ICs (26%) (Fig. 11). These findings suggested a correlation between free and complexed-IgG subclasses of anti-ADAMTS13 antibodies and did not support our hypothesis of a formation of ICs with a preference for certain IgG subclasses.

Due to the high prevalence of free and complexed IgG4 autoantibodies, we investigated the ability of the ADAMTS13-specific ICs to fix complement. This was evaluated using an ELISA that takes advantage of the specific binding of the complement subcomponent C1q to the Fc region of complexed IgG1-3. Circulating ICs binding to C1q were detected only in 6 out of 37 (16%) patients with TTP suggesting that the majority of the types of ICs detected in patients with TTP are not fixing complement. It remains possible though, that complement-fixing ICs did form but could not be detected because of their rapid deposition in tissues.

## *Inverse correlation of free and IC-sequestered anti-ADAMTS13 antibodies in a patient with acquired TTP*

We also analyzed the anti-ADAMTS13 antibody response and the concomitant appearance of circulating ICs during treatment of a patient with acquired TTP who died at day 64 after admission due to treatment refractoriness. This patient tested positive for the 3 classes of anti-ADAMTS13 antibodies with IgG1 as the main IgG subtype. By Co-IP, we detected circulating IgG-, IgA- and IgM-ICs despite daily PEX therapy. Interestingly, the ICs followed an inverse kinetics to the measured free antibody titers, becoming apparently undetectable when the titers of the free antibodies and inhibitor activity rose. These data strongly suggest that samples from acquired TTP patients need to be analyzed not only for free but also for complexed anti-ADAMTS13 antibodies to obtain a full picture of the status of the disease.

The IC ELISA revealed that for this patient the classes and subclasses of the immunoglobulin fraction forming the ICs correlated with those of the detected free antibodies. The patient had an IgG1-predominant immune response with detectable free and complexed-IgG1 antibodies and no detectable IgG4 (free or complexed) antibodies. These findings may be responsible, at least in part, for the treatment refractoriness and fatal outcome for this patient.

Interestingly, free ADAMTS13 antigen was not detected in most samples by our in-house ELISA whereas circulating ICs could be demonstrated by Co-IP and ELISA, indicating that ADAMTS13, either newly synthesized or exogenously administered by plasma infusion during PEX, was quantitatively sequestered by IC-formation. This mechanism may play an important role in the final response to treatment and should be particularly considered in patients refractory to treatment. The combined data of this study strongly suggest that samples from acquired TTP patients need to be analyzed not only for free but also for complexed anti-ADAMTS13 antibodies to obtain a full picture of the status of the disease.

## *Interaction of human IgG4 with rabbit IgG*

A sequential set of experiments, aimed initially to assess the origin of undesired background signals in the ADAMS13-IgG4-specific IC ELISA, revealed the unexpected fact that human IgG4 (but not IgG1-3) antibodies specifically bind to the Fc region of rabbit IgG antibodies. Publications describing the binding of human IgG4 to IgG antibodies of different animal species (including rabbit) came out after our experiments were performed[171;172]. Ito *et al*[171] showed that human IgG4 antibodies strongly bind to mouse, rabbit, guinea pig, bovine and goat IgG antibodies, but do not bind to sheep, horse and rat IgG. Interactions between human IgG4 and animal IgGs should therefore be taken into account when a new assay is designed because they are a potential source of high background and interferences.

## *Potential roles of anti-ADAMTS13 antibodies of the IgG4 and IgG1 subtypes and ADAMTS13-specific ICs in the pathogenesis of acquired TTP*

The relatively high incidence of IgG4 anti-ADAMTS13 antibodies and IgG4-containing ADAMTS13-specific ICs is a novel and rather unexpected finding, as association of IgG4 antibodies with direct pathologic effects are described in only a few diseases including pemphigus[173], sclerosing autoimmune pancreatitis and IgG4-related diseases[174]. IgG4 antibodies are thought to be functionally monovalent and non-cross-linking antibodies[164] through a process described as "Fab-arm exchange of IgG4 half-molecules", in which a heavy-light chain pair of one IgG4 molecule joins with another, unrelated, IgG4 half molecule, leading to a newly combined IgG4 molecule with two different antigen-binding sites[175]. Such bi-specific molecules are unable to crosslink antigen and, consequently, only form small and relatively harmless ICs with a low potential for induction of immune activation. Furthermore, IgG4 fails to activate potentially dangerous effector mechanisms; it has low affinity for complement C1q, which is required for IC-binding to endothelial cells and the initiation of the classical complement cascade[176], and binds to cellular FcγRs with less efficiency than the other IgG subclasses[156].

Moreover, the Fc region of human IgG4 antibodies can interact with its respective counterpart in other human IgG4 molecules[177]. This phenomenon may contribute in vivo to an enhancement of the antigen binding capacity (avidity) of IgG4, thereby optimizing IgG4-derived responses and maybe, in the case of autoantibodies, to a pathogenic effect.

A reduced number of patients presented with a predominant IgG1 response. In these patients the formation of high levels of IgG1-ICs may mediate more severe effector functions. IgG1 is known to have the potential to bind complement C1q and to activate cellular FcγRs[156]. Circulating IgG1-ICs can lead to endothelial cell activation, promoting inflammation and a pro-adhesive state, thus probably carrying a higher pathogenic potential when compared to IgG4-ICs. Furthermore, when present, IgA antibodies and IgA-ICs may also contribute to severity of the pathogenesis, because they have been shown to activate complement via the mannan-binding lectin pathway[178] and immune cells when binding to FcαRs[179], favoring an enhancement of complement-mediated inflammation and tissue damage.

Although anti-ADAMTS13 IgG4 antibodies have yet to be shown to be functionally monovalent and to interfere with complement activation *in vivo*, it is tempting to speculate that IgG4 autoantibodies, to some extent, act as "protective" antibodies in TTP patients, inducing a milder and treatable form of TTP, whereas IgG1 (and IgA) anti-ADAMTS13 antibodies have a higher pathogenic potential due to IC-related effector functions.

Even though our study is limited by the number of patients, and further studies are needed, we observed that patients are less likely to survive their first TTP event (four of seven patients died) if they have IgG1 and very low or undetectable IgG4 levels plus higher titers of other classes of anti-ADAMTS13 antibodies (particularly IgA antibodies), maybe due to formation of harmful ICs by these subclasses of antibodies. Similar observations were reported recently[161], where the presence of IgG1, IgG3 and IgA anti-ADAMTS13 antibodies in acute phase were associated with clinical severity and in the particular case of IgA antibodies, also with mortality.

The presence of increased levels of circulating ADAMTS13-specific ICs is likely to contribute to the pathogenic mechanisms leading to the onset of acquired TTP. Elevated levels of ICs are the main reason for systemic inflammatory manifestations associated with autoimmune diseases. Under normal conditions, ICs are quickly cleared by the reticuloendothelial system, but their continuous formation exceeds the clearance capacity of the system and the ICs build up in the circulation leading to endothelial cell activation and inflammation. The continuous presence of excessive amounts of circulating ICs might perpetuate a pro-inflammatory state promoting thrombosis and predisposing to relapse.

Furthermore, as described for SLE[180], ICs can also bind to B-cell receptors of auto-reactive B-cells resulting in signals leading to B-cell activation, proliferation and differentiation into autoantibody-producing cells. This activating cycle might cause formation of more autoantibodies and thus more ICs leading to progression of a deleterious effect.

While the amounts of circulating ICs should correlate with disease severity and activity, their quantification in plasma samples needs to consider several points: (i) the detected types of ICs may be irrelevant because harmful ICs could have already been deposited in tissues; (ii) the concentration of antigen, antibody and as a consequence ICs can change continuously during a chronic process, thus pathogenic ICs can form and deposit in a short period of time; (iii) the formation and clearance of ICs may not be in a steady state; and (iv) the setup of the assays does not allow discriminating between harmful and harmless ICs. Nonetheless, we believe that the detection and characterization of circulating ICs in patients with TTP will seed light onto the possible patho-mechanisms underlying TTP development. Whether such data are also of use for clinical monitoring, however, remains to be seen.

## *Prognostic marker for acquired TTP*

Beyond the characterization and elucidation of the role of anti-ADAMTS13 antibodies in the pathogenesis of TTP, the identification of prognostic factors during the first acute episode would be of crucial importance for making decisions in the clinic. TTP is a severe disease and its acute events may be life-threatening in the absence of fast and appropriate treatment. In addition, relapse occurs in 30-50% of the patients who survive an initial episode of TTP, being more often during the first year after the onset[118;181]. However, identifying prognostic factors for both short-term and long-term outcome still remains very difficult considering the broad heterogeneity of patients with TTP. This heterogeneity includes the clinical background (idiopathic versus disease-associated TTP, sporadic versus recurrent TTP) and the ADAMTS13-specific parameters (undetectable versus detectable ADAMTS13 activity or antigen, presence versus absence of ADAMTS13 inhibitor).

Several studies have investigated the significance of ADAMTS13 activity and inhibitors levels to predict outcomes. Most concluded that severe ADAMTS13 deficiency in combination with the presence of antibodies against ADAMTS13 either at presentation and/or during clinical remission are associated with a higher risk of disease recurrence[122;123;182-186].

We also have sought for prognostic factors that may help identifying patients at risk. We observed that anti-ADAMTS13 antibodies of the IgG class together with a high inhibitor titer at presentation were associated with persistence of undetectable ADAMTS13 activity in clinical remission (Fig. 6). Moreover, we were the first to investigate the possibility of an association between IgG subclasses and relapse, and found that high levels of IgG4 with undetectable IgG1 were statistically significantly associated with a trend towards recurrence of TTP. This suggests that high levels of IgG4 could help to identify patients who are at risk of recurrence and could be used, in association with ADAMTS13 activity and inhibitors, as a prognostic marker to predict possible relapse.

## 6- CONCLUSIONS

The pathophysiology of acute acquired TTP is characterized by severe deficiency of ADAMTS13 (activity and antigen) due to the presence of different classes (IgG, IgM and IgA) and subclasses (mainly IgG4 and IgG1) of inhibiting anti-ADAMTS13 antibodies. An immune response characterized by high levels of IgG4 predicts, at least partially, a more treatable form of TTP than if IgG1 antibodies are present. Antibodies against ADAMTS13 are also involved in immune-complex formation (mainly IgG4-containing immune complexes). Immune complexes might contribute to ADAMTS13 depletion from the circulation and probably to organ damage due to tissue deposition.

Measurement of inhibitory activity; free anti-ADAMTS13 antibodies as well as ADAMTS13-specific circulating ICs should be performed in patients presenting with acute acquired TTP. This information will help to better understand the course of the disease, especially in cases of refractory patients which may benefit of a more aggressive therapy.

Levels of IgG4 autoantibodies could be a recurrent predicting biomarker, although prospective trials with well-characterized patients are needed to substantiate our preliminary observations. The contribution made by IgG4 antibodies and IgG4-ICs to the overall pathologic mechanism in acquired TTP needs further investigation. We believe that the results of this study contributed to a better understanding of the pathogenesis leading to acquired TTP and the prognostic markers here identified might help to recognize patients at risk of disease recurrence or having a poor prognosis.

# 7- REFERENCES

1. Porter S, Clark IM, Kevorkian L, Edwards DR. The ADAMTS metalloproteinases. Biochem.J. 2005;386:15-27.

2. Sporn LA, Marder VJ, Wagner DD. Inducible secretion of large, biologically potent von Willebrand factor multimers. Cell 1986;46:185-190.

3. Arnout J, Hoylaerts MF, Lijnen HR. Haemostasis. Handb.Exp.Pharmacol. 20061-41.

4. Gale AJ. Continuing education course: current understanding of hemostasis. Toxicol.Pathol. 2011;39:273-280.

5. Furie B, Furie BC. Mechanisms of thrombus formation. N.Engl.J.Med. 2008;359:938-949.

6. Ruggeri ZM. Platelet adhesion under flow. Microcirculation. 2009;16:58-83.

7. Andrews RK, Gardiner EE, Shen Y, Whisstock JC, Berndt MC. Glycoprotein Ib-IX-V. Int.J.Biochem.Cell Biol. 2003;35:1170-1174.

8. Ruggeri ZM, Mendolicchio GL. Adhesion mechanisms in platelet function. Circ.Res. 2007;100:1673-1685.

9. Savage B, Sixma JJ, Ruggeri ZM. Functional self-association of von Willebrand factor during platelet adhesion under flow. Proc.Natl.Acad.Sci.U.S.A 2002;99:425-430.

10. Dahlback B. Blood coagulation and its regulation by anticoagulant pathways: genetic pathogenesis of bleeding and thrombotic diseases. J.Intern.Med. 2005;257:209-223.

11. Jackson SP. The growing complexity of platelet aggregation. Blood 2007;109:5087-5095.

12. Tao L, Zhang Y, Xi X, Kieffer N. Recent advances in the understanding of the molecular mechanisms regulating platelet integrin alphaIIbbeta3 activation. Protein Cell 2010;1:627-637.

13. DAVIE EW, RATNOFF OD. Waterfall sequence for intrinsic blood clotting. Science 1964;145:1310-1312.

14. MACFARLANE RG. An enzyme cascade in the blood clotting mechanism, and its function as a biochemical amplifier. Nature 1964;202:498-499.

15. Butenas S, Orfeo T, Mann KG. Tissue factor in coagulation: Which? Where? When? Arterioscler.Thromb.Vasc.Biol. 2009;29:1989-1996.

16. Butenas S, Mann KG. Blood coagulation. Biochemistry (Mosc.) 2002;67:3-12.
17. Renne T, Gailani D. Role of Factor XII in hemostasis and thrombosis: clinical implications. Expert.Rev.Cardiovasc.Ther 2007;5:733-741.
18. Muller F, Renne T. Novel roles for factor XII-driven plasma contact activation system. Curr Opin Hematol. 2008;15:516-521.
19. Lorand L. Factor XIII: structure, activation, and interactions with fibrinogen and fibrin. Ann.N.Y.Acad.Sci. 2001;936:291-311.
20. Hoffman M. Remodeling the blood coagulation cascade. J.Thromb.Thrombolysis. 2003;16:17-20.
21. Monroe DM, Hoffman M. What does it take to make the perfect clot? Arterioscler.Thromb.Vasc.Biol. 2006;26:41-48.
22. Terraube V, O'Donnell JS, Jenkins PV. Factor VIII and von Willebrand factor interaction: biological, clinical and therapeutic importance. Haemophilia. 2010;16:3-13.
23. Nachman R, Levine R, Jaffe EA. Synthesis of factor VIII antigen by cultured guinea pig megakaryocytes. J.Clin.Invest 1977;60:914-921.
24. Jaffe EA, Hoyer LW, Nachman RL. Synthesis of von Willebrand factor by cultured human endothelial cells. Proc.Natl.Acad.Sci.U.S.A 1974;71:1906-1909.
25. Wagner DD. Cell biology of von Willebrand factor. Annu.Rev.Cell Biol. 1990;6:217-246.
26. Sadler JE. Biochemistry and genetics of von Willebrand factor. Annu.Rev.Biochem. 1998;67:395-424.
27. Giblin JP, Hewlett LJ, Hannah MJ. Basal secretion of von Willebrand factor from human endothelial cells. Blood 2008;112:957-964.
28. Sporn LA, Chavin SI, Marder VJ, Wagner DD. Biosynthesis of von Willebrand protein by human megakaryocytes. J.Clin.Invest 1985;76:1102-1106.
29. Moake JL, Turner NA, Stathopoulos NA, Nolasco LH, Hellums JD. Involvement of large plasma von Willebrand factor (vWF) multimers and unusually large vWF forms derived from endothelial cells in shear stress-induced platelet aggregation. J.Clin.Invest 1986;78:1456-1461.

30. Furlan M, Robles R, Lämmle B. Partial purification and characterization of a protease from human plasma cleaving von Willebrand factor to fragments produced by in vivo proteolysis. Blood 1996;87:4223-4234.

31. Tsai HM. Physiologic cleavage of von Willebrand factor by a plasma protease is dependent on its conformation and requires calcium ion. Blood 1996;87:4235-4244.

32. Moake JL, Rudy CK, Troll JH et al. Unusually large plasma factor VIII:von Willebrand factor multimers in chronic relapsing thrombotic thrombocytopenic purpura. N.Engl.J.Med. 1982;307:1432-1435.

33. Sadler JE, Budde U, Eikenboom JC et al. Update on the pathophysiology and classification of von Willebrand disease: a report of the Subcommittee on von Willebrand Factor. J Thromb Haemost. 2006;4:2103-2114.

34. Furlan M, Robles R, Solenthaler M et al. Deficient activity of von Willebrand factor-cleaving protease in chronic relapsing thrombotic thrombocytopenic purpura. Blood 1997;89:3097-3103.

35. Furlan M, Robles R, Galbusera M et al. von Willebrand factor-cleaving protease in thrombotic thrombocytopenic purpura and the hemolytic-uremic syndrome. N.Engl.J.Med. 1998;339:1578-1584.

36. Tsai HM, Lian EC. Antibodies to von Willebrand factor-cleaving protease in acute thrombotic thrombocytopenic purpura. N.Engl.J.Med. 1998;339:1585-1594.

37. Gerritsen HE, Robles R, Lämmle B, Furlan M. Partial amino acid sequence of purified von Willebrand factor-cleaving protease. Blood 2001;98:1654-1661.

38. Fujikawa K, Suzuki H, McMullen B, Chung D. Purification of human von Willebrand factor-cleaving protease and its identification as a new member of the metalloproteinase family. Blood 2001;98:1662-1666.

39. Soejima K, Mimura N, Hirashima M et al. A novel human metalloprotease synthesized in the liver and secreted into the blood: possibly, the von Willebrand factor-cleaving protease? J.Biochem. 2001;130:475-480.

40. Zheng X, Chung D, Takayama TK et al. Structure of von Willebrand factor-cleaving protease (ADAMTS13), a metalloprotease involved in thrombotic thrombocytopenic purpura. J.Biol.Chem. 2001;276:41059-41063.

41. Levy GG, Nichols WC, Lian EC et al. Mutations in a member of the ADAMTS gene family cause thrombotic thrombocytopenic purpura. Nature 2001;413:488-494.

42. Plaimauer B, Zimmermann K, Volkel D et al. Cloning, expression, and functional characterization of the von Willebrand factor-cleaving protease (ADAMTS13). Blood 2002;100:3626-3632.

43. Uemura M, Tatsumi K, Matsumoto M et al. Localization of ADAMTS13 to the stellate cells of human liver. Blood 2005;106:922-924.

44. Zhou W, Inada M, Lee TP et al. ADAMTS13 is expressed in hepatic stellate cells. Lab Invest 2005;85:780-788.

45. Suzuki M, Murata M, Matsubara Y et al. Detection of von Willebrand factor-cleaving protease (ADAMTS-13) in human platelets. Biochem.Biophys.Res.Commun. 2004;313:212-216.

46. Turner N, Nolasco L, Tao Z, Dong JF, Moake J. Human endothelial cells synthesize and release ADAMTS-13. J.Thromb.Haemost. 2006;4:1396-1404.

47. Manea M, Kristoffersson A, Schneppenheim R et al. Podocytes express ADAMTS13 in normal renal cortex and in patients with thrombotic thrombocytopenic purpura. Br.J.Haematol. 2007;138:651-662.

48. Manea M, Tati R, Karlsson J, Bekassy ZD, Karpman D. Biologically active ADAMTS13 is expressed in renal tubular epithelial cells. Pediatr.Nephrol. 2010;25:87-96.

49. Majerus EM, Zheng X, Tuley EA, Sadler JE. Cleavage of the ADAMTS13 propeptide is not required for protease activity. J.Biol.Chem. 2003;278:46643-46648.

50. Furlan M, Robles R, Morselli B, Sandoz P, Lämmle B. Recovery and half-life of von Willebrand factor-cleaving protease after plasma therapy in patients with thrombotic thrombocytopenic purpura. Thromb.Haemost. 1999;81:8-13.

51. Rieger M, Ferrari S, Kremer Hovinga JA et al. Relation between ADAMTS13 activity and ADAMTS13 antigen levels in healthy donors and patients with thrombotic microangiopathies (TMA). Thromb Haemost. 2006;95:212-220.

52. Feys HB, Anderson PJ, Vanhoorelbeke K, Majerus EM, Sadler JE. Multi-step binding of ADAMTS-13 to von Willebrand factor. J.Thromb.Haemost. 2009;7:2088-2095.

53. Soejima K, Nakamura H, Hirashima M et al. Analysis on the molecular species and concentration of circulating ADAMTS13 in Blood. J.Biochem. 2006;139:147-154.

54. Zhou W, Tsai HM. N-Glycans of ADAMTS13 modulate its secretion and von Willebrand factor cleaving activity. Blood 2009;113:929-935.

55. Ricketts LM, Dlugosz M, Luther KB, Haltiwanger RS, Majerus EM. O-fucosylation is required for ADAMTS13 secretion. J.Biol.Chem. 2007;282:17014-17023.

56. Hiura H, Matsui T, Matsumoto M et al. Proteolytic fragmentation and sugar chains of plasma ADAMTS13 purified by a conformation-dependent monoclonal antibody. J.Biochem. 2010;148:403-411.

57. Crawley JT, Lam JK, Rance JB et al. Proteolytic inactivation of ADAMTS13 by thrombin and plasmin. Blood 2005;105:1085-1093.

58. Akiyama M, Takeda S, Kokame K, Takagi J, Miyata T. Crystal structures of the noncatalytic domains of ADAMTS13 reveal multiple discontinuous exosites for von Willebrand factor. Proc.Natl.Acad.Sci.U.S.A 2009;106:19274-19279.

59. Bode W, Fernandez-Catalan C, Tschesche H et al. Structural properties of matrix metalloproteinases. Cell Mol.Life Sci. 1999;55:639-652.

60. Gardner MD, Chion CK, de GR et al. A functional calcium-binding site in the metalloprotease domain of ADAMTS13. Blood 2009;113:1149-1157.

61. Davis AK, Makar RS, Stowell CP, Kuter DJ, Dzik WH. ADAMTS13 binds to CD36: a potential mechanism for platelet and endothelial localization of ADAMTS13. Transfusion 2009;49:206-213.

62. Shang D, Zheng XW, Niiya M, Zheng XL. Apical sorting of ADAMTS13 in vascular endothelial cells and Madin-Darby canine kidney cells depends on the CUB domains and their association with lipid rafts. Blood 2006;108:2207-2215.

63. Tao Z, Peng Y, Nolasco L et al. Recombinant CUB-1 domain polypeptide inhibits the cleavage of ULVWF strings by ADAMTS13 under flow conditions. Blood 2005;106:4139-4145.

64. Zhang P, Pan W, Rux AH, Sachais BS, Zheng XL. The cooperative activity between the carboxyl-terminal TSP1 repeats and the CUB domains of ADAMTS13 is crucial for recognition of von Willebrand factor under flow. Blood 2007;110:1887-1894.

65. Zhou Z, Yeh HC, Jing H et al. Cysteine residues in CUB-1 domain are critical for ADAMTS13 secretion and stability. Thromb.Haemost. 2011;105:21-30.

66. Zhang Q, Zhou YF, Zhang CZ et al. Structural specializations of A2, a force-sensing domain in the ultralarge vascular protein von Willebrand factor. Proc.Natl.Acad.Sci.U.S.A 2009;106:9226-9231.

67. Padilla A, Moake JL, Bernardo A et al. P-selectin anchors newly released ultralarge von Willebrand factor multimers to the endothelial cell surface. Blood 2004;103:2150-2156.

68. Huang J, Roth R, Heuser JE, Sadler JE. Integrin alpha(v)beta(3) on human endothelial cells binds von Willebrand factor strings under fluid shear stress. Blood 2009;113:1589-1597.

69. Turner NA, Nolasco L, Ruggeri ZM, Moake JL. Endothelial cell ADAMTS-13 and VWF: production, release, and VWF string cleavage. Blood 2009;114:5102-5111.

70. Jin SY, Skipwith CG, Shang D, Zheng XL. von Willebrand factor cleaved from endothelial cells by ADAMTS13 remains ultralarge in size. J Thromb Haemost 2009;7:1749-1752.

71. Dong JF, Moake JL, Nolasco L et al. ADAMTS-13 rapidly cleaves newly secreted ultralarge von Willebrand factor multimers on the endothelial surface under flowing conditions. Blood 2002;100:4033-4039.

72. Dong JF, Whitelock J, Bernardo A, Ball C, Cruz MA. Variations among normal individuals in the cleavage of endothelial-derived ultra-large von Willebrand factor under flow. J.Thromb.Haemost. 2004;2:1460-1466.

73. Yeh HC, Zhou Z, Choi H et al. Disulfide bond reduction of von Willebrand factor by ADAMTS-13. J.Thromb.Haemost. 2010;8:2778-2788.

74. Anderson PJ, Kokame K, Sadler JE. Zinc and calcium ions cooperatively modulate ADAMTS13 activity. J.Biol.Chem. 2006;281:850-857.

75. Shim K, Anderson PJ, Tuley EA, Wiswall E, Sadler JE. Platelet-VWF complexes are preferred substrates of ADAMTS13 under fluid shear stress. Blood 2008;111:651-657.

76. Cao W, Krishnaswamy S, Camire RM, Lenting PJ, Zheng XL. Factor VIII accelerates proteolytic cleavage of von Willebrand factor by ADAMTS13. Proc.Natl.Acad.Sci.U.S.A 2008;105:7416-7421.

77. Skipwith CG, Cao W, Zheng XL. Factor VIII and platelets synergistically accelerate cleavage of von Willebrand factor by ADAMTS13 under fluid shear stress. J.Biol.Chem. 2010;285:28596-28603.

78. De Cristofaro R, Peyvandi F, Palla R et al. Role of chloride ions in modulation of the interaction between von Willebrand factor and ADAMTS-13. J.Biol.Chem. 2005;280:23295-23302.

79. De Cristofaro R, Peyvandi F, Baronciani L et al. Molecular mapping of the chloride-binding site in von Willebrand factor (VWF): energetics and

conformational effects on the VWF/ADAMTS-13 interaction. J Biol Chem 2006;281:30400-30411.

80. Chen J, Fu X, Wang Y et al. Oxidative modification of von Willebrand factor by neutrophil oxidants inhibits its cleavage by ADAMTS13. Blood 2010;115:706-712.

81. Lancellotti S, De F, V, Pozzi N et al. Formation of methionine sulfoxide by peroxynitrite at position 1606 of von Willebrand factor inhibits its cleavage by ADAMTS-13: A new prothrombotic mechanism in diseases associated with oxidative stress. Free Radic.Biol.Med. 2010;48:446-456.

82. Zheng X, Nishio K, Majerus EM, Sadler JE. Cleavage of von Willebrand factor requires the spacer domain of the metalloprotease ADAMTS13. J.Biol.Chem. 2003;278:30136-30141.

83. Ai J, Smith P, Wang S, Zhang P, Zheng XL. The proximal carboxyl-terminal domains of ADAMTS13 determine substrate specificity and are all required for cleavage of von Willebrand factor. J Biol Chem 2005;280:29428-29434.

84. Gao W, Anderson PJ, Majerus EM, Tuley EA, Sadler JE. Exosite interactions contribute to tension-induced cleavage of von Willebrand factor by the antithrombotic ADAMTS13 metalloprotease. Proc.Natl.Acad.Sci.U.S.A 2006;103:19099-19104.

85. Tao Z, Wang Y, Choi H et al. Cleavage of ultralarge multimers of von Willebrand factor by C-terminal-truncated mutants of ADAMTS-13 under flow. Blood 2005;106:141-143.

86. Kokame K, Matsumoto M, Fujimura Y, Miyata T. VWF73, a region from D1596 to R1668 of von Willebrand factor, provides a minimal substrate for ADAMTS-13. Blood 2004;103:607-612.

87. Gao W, Anderson PJ, Sadler JE. Extensive contacts between ADAMTS13 exosites and von Willebrand factor domain A2 contribute to substrate specificity. Blood 2008;112:1713-1719.

88. Jin SY, Skipwith CG, Zheng XL. Amino acid residues Arg659, Arg660 and Tyr661 in the spacer domain of ADAMTS13 are critical for cleavage of von Willebrand factor. Blood 2010;115:2300-2310.

89. Pos W, Crawley JT, Fijnheer R et al. An autoantibody epitope comprising residues R660, Y661, and Y665 in the ADAMTS13 spacer domain identifies a binding site for the A2 domain of VWF. Blood 2010;115:1640-1649.

90. de Groot R., Bardhan A, Ramroop N, Lane DA, Crawley JT. Essential role of the disintegrin-like domain in ADAMTS13 function. Blood 2009;113:5609-5616.

91. de Groot R., Lane DA, Crawley JT. The ADAMTS13 metalloprotease domain: roles of subsites in enzyme activity and specificity. Blood 2010;116:3064-3072.

92. Majerus EM, Anderson PJ, Sadler JE. Binding of ADAMTS13 to von Willebrand factor. J.Biol.Chem. 2005;280:21773-21778.

93. Banno F, Chauhan AK, Kokame K et al. The distal carboxyl-terminal domains of ADAMTS13 are required for regulation of in vivo thrombus formation. Blood 2009;113:5323-5329.

94. De Maeyer B, De Meyer SF, Feys HB et al. The distal carboxyterminal domains of murine ADAMTS13 influence proteolysis of platelet-decorated VWF strings in vivo. J.Thromb.Haemost. 2010;8:2305-2312.

95. Gerritsen HE, Turecek PL, Schwarz HP, Lammle B, Furlan M. Assay of von Willebrand factor (vWF)-cleaving protease based on decreased collagen binding affinity of degraded vWF: a tool for the diagnosis of thrombotic thrombocytopenic purpura (TTP). Thromb.Haemost. 1999;82:1386-1389.

96. Obert B, Tout H, Veyradier A et al. Estimation of the von Willebrand factor-cleaving protease in plasma using monoclonal antibodies to vWF. Thromb.Haemost. 1999;82:1382-1385.

97. Böhm M, Vigh T, Scharrer I. Evaluation and clinical application of a new method for measuring activity of von Willebrand factor-cleaving metalloprotease (ADAMTS13). Ann.Hematol. 2002;81:430-435.

98. Cruz MA, Whitelock J, Dong JF. Evaluation of ADAMTS-13 activity in plasma using recombinant von Willebrand Factor A2 domain polypeptide as substrate. Thromb.Haemost. 2003;90:1204-1209.

99. Whitelock JL, Nolasco L, Bernardo A et al. ADAMTS-13 activity in plasma is rapidly measured by a new ELISA method that uses recombinant VWF-A2 domain as substrate. J.Thromb.Haemost. 2004;2:485-491.

100. Kokame K, Nobe Y, Kokubo Y, Okayama A, Miyata T. FRETS-VWF73, a first fluorogenic substrate for ADAMTS13 assay. Br.J Haematol. 2005;129:93-100.

101. Groot E, Hulstein JJ, Rison CN, de Groot PG, Fijnheer R. FRETS-VWF73: a rapid and predictive tool for thrombotic thrombocytopenic purpura. J.Thromb.Haemost. 2006;4:698-699.

102. Mahdian R, Rayes J, Girma JP et al. Comparison of FRETS-VWF73 to full-length VWF as a substrate for ADAMTS13 activity measurement in human plasma samples. Thromb Haemost. 2006;95:1049-1051.

103. Kremer Hovinga JA, Mottini M, Lammle B. Measurement of ADAMTS-13 activity in plasma by the FRETS-VWF73 assay: comparison with other assay methods. J.Thromb.Haemost. 2006;4:1146-1148.

104. Kasper CK, Aledort L, Aronson D et al. Proceedings: A more uniform measurement of factor VIII inhibitors. Thromb.Diath.Haemorrh. 1975;34:612.

105. Tripodi A, Chantarangkul V, Böhm M et al. Measurement of von Willebrand factor cleaving protease (ADAMTS-13): results of an international collaborative study involving 11 methods testing the same set of coded plasmas. J Thromb Haemost. 2004;2:1601-1609.

106. Han Y, Xiao J, Falls E, Zheng XL. A shear-based assay for assessing plasma ADAMTS13 activity and inhibitors in patients with thrombotic thrombocytopenic purpura. Transfusion 2011;51:1580-1591.

107. Feys HB, Liu F, Dong N et al. ADAMTS-13 plasma level determination uncovers antigen absence in acquired thrombotic thrombocytopenic purpura and ethnic differences. J.Thromb.Haemost. 2006;4:955-962.

108. Yagi H, Ito S, Kato S et al. Plasma levels of ADAMTS13 antigen determined with an enzyme immunoassay using a neutralizing monoclonal antibody parallel ADAMTS13 activity levels. Int.J.Hematol. 2007;85:403-407.

109. Tripodi A, Peyvandi F, Chantarangkul V et al. Second international collaborative study evaluating performance characteristics of methods measuring the von Willebrand factor cleaving protease (ADAMTS-13). J Thromb Haemost 2008;6:1534-1541.

110. Moake J. Thrombotic thrombocytopenia purpura (TTP) and other thrombotic microangiopathies. Best.Pract.Res.Clin.Haematol. 2009;22:567-576.

111. Copelovitch L, Kaplan BS. The thrombotic microangiopathies. Pediatr.Nephrol. 2008;23:1761-1767.

112. Benz K, Amann K. Thrombotic microangiopathy: new insights. Curr.Opin.Nephrol.Hypertens. 2010;19:242-247.

113. Moschcowitz E. Hyaline thrombosis of the terminal arterioles and capillaries: a hitherto undescribed disease. Proc.NY Pathol Soc 1924;24:21-24.

114. Moake JL. Thrombotic microangiopathies. N.Engl.J Med. 2002;347:589-600.

115. George JN. Clinical practice. Thrombotic thrombocytopenic purpura. N.Engl.J Med. 2006;354:1927-1935.

116. Rock GA, Shumak KH, Buskard NA et al. Comparison of plasma exchange with plasma infusion in the treatment of thrombotic thrombocytopenic purpura. Canadian Apheresis Study Group. N.Engl.J.Med. 1991;325:393-397.

117. Fontana S, Kremer Hovinga JA, Lammle B, Mansouri TB. Treatment of thrombotic thrombocytopenic purpura. Vox Sang. 2006;90:245-254.

118. George JN. The thrombotic thrombocytopenic purpura and hemolytic uremic syndromes: evaluation, management, and long-term outcomes experience of the Oklahoma TTP-HUS Registry, 1989-2007. Kidney Int.Suppl 2009S52-S54.

119. Terrell DR, Williams LA, Vesely SK et al. The incidence of thrombotic thrombocytopenic purpura-hemolytic uremic syndrome: all patients, idiopathic patients, and patients with severe ADAMTS-13 deficiency. J Thromb Haemost. 2005;3:1432-1436.

120. Scully M, Yarranton H, Liesner R et al. Regional UK TTP registry: correlation with laboratory ADAMTS 13 analysis and clinical features. Br.J Haematol. 2008;142:819-826.

121. Kokame K, Matsumoto M, Soejima K et al. Mutations and common polymorphisms in ADAMTS13 gene responsible for von Willebrand factor-cleaving protease activity. Proc.Natl.Acad.Sci.U.S.A 2002;99:11902-11907.

122. Zheng XL, Kaufman RM, Goodnough LT, Sadler JE. Effect of plasma exchange on plasma ADAMTS13 metalloprotease activity, inhibitor level, and clinical outcome in patients with idiopathic and nonidiopathic thrombotic thrombocytopenic purpura. Blood 2004;103:4043-4049.

123. Peyvandi F, Ferrari S, Lavoretano S, Canciani MT, Mannucci PM. von Willebrand factor cleaving protease (ADAMTS-13) and ADAMTS-13 neutralizing autoantibodies in 100 patients with thrombotic thrombocytopenic purpura. Br.J Haematol. 2004;127:433-439.

124. Zakarija A, Kwaan HC, Moake JL et al. Ticlopidine- and clopidogrel-associated thrombotic thrombocytopenic purpura (TTP): review of clinical, laboratory, epidemiological, and pharmacovigilance findings (1989-2008). Kidney Int Suppl 2009S20-S24.

125. Sadler JE. Thrombotic thrombocytopenic purpura: a moving target. Hematology.Am.Soc.Hematol.Educ.Program. 2006415-420.

126. Tsai HM. Pathophysiology of thrombotic thrombocytopenic purpura. Int.J.Hematol. 2010;91:1-19.

127. Lotta LA, Garagiola I, Palla R, Cairo A, Peyvandi F. ADAMTS13 mutations and polymorphisms in congenital thrombotic thrombocytopenic purpura. Hum.Mutat. 2010;31:11-19.

128. Plaimauer B, Fuhrmann J, Mohr G et al. Modulation of ADAMTS13 secretion and specific activity by a combination of common amino acid polymorphisms and a missense mutation. Blood 2006;107:118-125.

129. George JN. Congenital thrombotic thrombocytopenic purpura: Lessons for recognition and management of rare syndromes. Pediatr.Blood Cancer 2008;50:947-948.

130. Scheiflinger F, Knöbl P, Trattner B et al. Nonneutralizing IgM and IgG antibodies to von Willebrand factor-cleaving protease (ADAMTS-13) in a patient with thrombotic thrombocytopenic purpura. Blood 2003;102:3241-3243.

131. Shelat SG, Smith P, Ai J, Zheng XL. Inhibitory autoantibodies against ADAMTS-13 in patients with thrombotic thrombocytopenic purpura bind ADAMTS-13 protease and may accelerate its clearance in vivo. J Thromb Haemost. 2006;4:1707-1717.

132. Rieger M, Mannucci PM, Kremer Hovinga JA et al. ADAMTS13 autoantibodies in patients with thrombotic microangiopathies and other immunomediated diseases. Blood 2005;106:1262-1267.

133. Tsai HM, Raoufi M, Zhou W et al. ADAMTS13-binding IgG are present in patients with thrombotic thrombocytopenic purpura. Thromb Haemost. 2006;95:886-892.

134. Klaus C, Plaimauer B, Studt JD et al. Epitope mapping of ADAMTS13 autoantibodies in acquired thrombotic thrombocytopenic purpura. Blood 2004;103:4514-4519.

135. Luken BM, Turenhout EA, Hulstein JJ et al. The spacer domain of ADAMTS13 contains a major binding site for antibodies in patients with thrombotic thrombocytopenic purpura. Thromb Haemost. 2005;93:267-274.

136. Pos W, Sorvillo N, Fijnheer R et al. Residues Arg568 and Phe592 contribute to an antigenic surface for anti-ADAMTS13 antibodies in the spacer domain. Haematologica 2011;96:1670-1677.

137. Zheng XL, Wu HM, Shang D et al. Multiple domains of ADAMTS13 are targeted by autoantibodies against ADAMTS13 in patients with acquired idiopathic thrombotic thrombocytopenic purpura. Haematologica 2010;95:1555-1562.

138. Coppo P, Busson M, Veyradier A et al. HLA-DRB1*11: a strong risk factor for acquired severe ADAMTS13 deficiency-related idiopathic thrombotic thrombocytopenic purpura in Caucasians. J Thromb Haemost 2010;8:856-859.

139. Scully M, Brown J, Patel R et al. Human leukocyte antigen association in idiopathic thrombotic thrombocytopenic purpura: evidence for an immunogenetic link. J Thromb Haemost 2010;8:257-262.

140. Nguyen L, Terrell DR, Duvall D, Vesely SK, George JN. Complications of plasma exchange in patients treated for thrombotic thrombocytopenic purpura. IV. An additional study of 43 consecutive patients, 2005 to 2008. Transfusion 2009;49:392-394.

141. Elliott MA, Heit JA, Pruthi RK et al. Rituximab for refractory and or relapsing thrombotic thrombocytopenic purpura related to immune-mediated severe ADAMTS13-deficiency: a report of four cases and a systematic review of the literature. Eur.J.Haematol. 2009;83:365-372.

142. Dubois L, Gray DK. Case series: splenectomy: does it still play a role in the management of thrombotic thrombocytopenic purpura? Can.J.Surg. 2010;53:349-355.

143. Silverstein RL, Febbraio M. CD36, a scavenger receptor involved in immunity, metabolism, angiogenesis, and behavior. Sci.Signal. 2009;2:re3.

144. Febbraio M, Silverstein RL. CD36: implications in cardiovascular disease. Int.J.Biochem.Cell Biol. 2007;39:2012-2030.

145. Rac ME, Safranow K, Poncyljusz W. Molecular basis of human CD36 gene mutations. Mol.Med. 2007;13:288-296.

146. Yamamoto N, Ikeda H, Tandon NN et al. A platelet membrane glycoprotein (GP) deficiency in healthy blood donors: Naka- platelets lack detectable GPIV (CD36). Blood 1990;76:1698-1703.

147. Saw CL, Szykoluk H, Curtis BR et al. Two cases of platelet transfusion refractoriness associated with anti-CD36. Transfusion 2010;50:2638-2642.

148. Tandon NN, Rock G, Jamieson GA. Anti-CD36 antibodies in thrombotic thrombocytopenic purpura. Br.J.Haematol. 1994;88:816-825.

149. Schultz DR, Arnold PI, Jy W et al. Anti-CD36 autoantibodies in thrombotic thrombocytopenic purpura and other thrombotic disorders: identification of an 85 kD form of CD36 as a target antigen. Br.J.Haematol. 1998;103:849-857.

150. Wright JF, Wang H, Hornstein A et al. Characterization of platelet glycoproteins and platelet/endothelial cell antibodies in patients with thrombotic thrombocytopenic purpura. Br.J.Haematol. 1999;107:546-555.

151. al-Shahi R, Mason JC, Rao R et al. Systemic lupus erythematosus, thrombocytopenia, microangiopathic haemolytic anaemia and anti-CD36 antibodies. Br.J.Rheumatol. 1997;36:794-798.

152. Pelegri Y, Cerrato G, Martinuzzo ME, Carreras LO, Forastiero RR. Link between anti-CD36 antibodies and thrombosis in the antiphospholipid syndrome. Clin.Exp.Rheumatol. 2003;21:221-224.

153. Rock G, Anderson D, Clark W et al. Does cryosupernatant plasma improve outcome in thrombotic thrombocytopenic purpura? No answer yet. Br.J.Haematol. 2005;129:79-86.

154. Studt JD, Kremer Hovinga JA, Alberio L, Bianchi V, Lämmle B. Von Willebrand factor-cleaving protease (ADAMTS-13) activity in thrombotic microangiopathies: diagnostic experience 2001/2002 of a single research laboratory. Swiss.Med.Wkly. 2003;133:325-332.

155. Veyradier A, Obert B, Houllier A, Meyer D, Girma JP. Specific von Willebrand factor-cleaving protease in thrombotic microangiopathies: a study of 111 cases. Blood 2001;98:1765-1772.

156. Jefferis R, Pound J, Lund J, Goodall M. Effector mechanisms activated by human IgG subclass antibodies: clinical and molecular aspects. Ann.Biol.Clin.(Paris) 1994;52:57-65.

157. Stavnezer J. Immunoglobulin class switching. Curr Opin Immunol 1996;8:199-205.

158. Iwata Y, Komura K, Kodera M et al. Correlation of IgE autoantibody to BP180 with a severe form of bullous pemphigoid. Arch.Dermatol. 2008;144:41-48.

159. Atta AM, Santiago MB, Guerra FG, Pereira MM, Sousa Atta ML. Autoimmune response of IgE antibodies to cellular self-antigens in systemic Lupus Erythematosus. Int.Arch.Allergy Immunol. 2010;152:401-406.

160. Ferrari S, Scheiflinger F, Rieger M et al. Prognostic value of anti-ADAMTS 13 antibody features (Ig isotype, titer, and inhibitory effect) in a cohort of 35 adult French patients undergoing a first episode of thrombotic microangiopathy with undetectable ADAMTS 13 activity. Blood 2007;109:2815-2822.

161. Bettoni, G, Palla, R., Valsecchi, C., Consonni, D, Trisolini, S, Carbone, C, and Peyvandi, F. ADAMTS13 activity and autoantibodies classes and subclasses as prognostic predictors in acquired thrombotic thrombocytopenic purpura (TTP). Poster presented at the 7th Bari International Conference, Italy. 2011. Ref Type: Pamphlet

162. Wilson WA, Faghiri Z, Taheri F, Gharavi AE. Significance of IgA antiphospholipid antibodies. Lupus 1998;7 Suppl 2:S110-S113.

163. Shen YM, Lee R, Frenkel E, Sarode R. IgA antiphospholipid antibodies are an independent risk factor for thromboses. Lupus 2008;17:996-1003.

164. Aalberse RC, Stapel SO, Schuurman J, Rispens T. Immunoglobulin G4: an odd antibody. Clin.Exp.Allergy 2009;39:469-477.

165. Mayadas TN, Tsokos GC, Tsuboi N. Mechanisms of immune complex-mediated neutrophil recruitment and tissue injury. Circulation 2009;120:2012-2024.

166. Bayer AS, Theofilopoulos AN, Eisenberg R, Friedman SG, Guze LB. Thrombotic thrombocytopenic purpura-like syndrome associated with infective endocarditis. A possible immune complex disorder. JAMA 1977;238:408-410.

167. Bukowski RM, King JW, Hewlett JS. Plasmapheresis in the treatment of thrombotic thrombocytopenic purpura. Blood 1977;50:413-417.

168. Celada A, Perrin LH. Circulating immune complexes in thrombotic thrombocytopenic purpura (TTP). Blood 1978;52:855.

169. Neame PB, Hirsh J. Circulating immune complexes in thrombotic thrombocytopenic purpura (TTP). Blood 1978;51:559-560.

170. Yang S, Jin M, Lin S, Cataland SR, Wu HM. ADAMTS13 activity and antigen during therapy and follow-up of patients with idiopathic thrombotic thrombocytopenic purpura: correlation with clinical outcome. Haematologica 2011;96:1521-1527.

171. Ito T, Kitahara K, Umemura T et al. A novel heterophilic antibody interaction involves IgG4. Scand.J.Immunol. 2010;71:109-114.

172. Rispens T, Leeuwen A, Vennegoor A et al. Measurement of serum levels of natalizumab, an immunoglobulin G4 therapeutic monoclonal antibody. Anal.Biochem. 2011;411:271-276.

173. Mihai S, Chiriac MT, Herrero-Gonzalez JE et al. IgG4 autoantibodies induce dermal-epidermal separation. J.Cell Mol.Med. 2007;11:1117-1128.

174. Okazaki K, Uchida K, Koyabu M, Miyoshi H, Takaoka M. Recent advances in the concept and diagnosis of autoimmune pancreatitis and IgG4-related disease. J.Gastroenterol. 2011;46:277-288.

175. van der Neut KM, Schuurman J, Losen M et al. Anti-inflammatory activity of human IgG4 antibodies by dynamic Fab arm exchange. Science 2007;317:1554-1557.

176. Stokol T, O'Donnell P, Xiao L et al. C1q governs deposition of circulating immune complexes and leukocyte Fcgamma receptors mediate subsequent neutrophil recruitment. J.Exp.Med. 2004;200:835-846.

177. Rispens T, Ooievaar-De HP, Vermeulen E et al. Human IgG4 binds to IgG4 and conformationally altered IgG1 via Fc-Fc interactions. J.Immunol. 2009;182:4275-4281.

178. Roos A, Bouwman LH, van Gijlswijk-Janssen DJ et al. Human IgA activates the complement system via the mannan-binding lectin pathway. J.Immunol. 2001;167:2861-2868.

179. Monteiro RC. Role of IgA and IgA fc receptors in inflammation. J.Clin.Immunol. 2010;30:1-9.

180. Chiang EY, Yu X, Grogan JL. Immune complex-mediated cell activation from systemic lupus erythematosus and rheumatoid arthritis patients elaborate different requirements for IRAK1/4 kinase activity across human cell types. J.Immunol. 2011;186:1279-1288.

181. Willis MS, Bandarenko N. Relapse of thrombotic thrombocytopenic purpura: is it a continuum of disease? Semin.Thromb.Hemost. 2005;31:700-708.

182. Vesely SK, George JN, Lammle B et al. ADAMTS13 activity in thrombotic thrombocytopenic purpura-hemolytic uremic syndrome: relation to presenting features and clinical outcomes in a prospective cohort of 142 patients. Blood 2003;102:60-68.

183. Raife T, Atkinson B, Montgomery R, Vesely S, Friedman K. Severe deficiency of VWF-cleaving protease (ADAMTS13) activity defines a distinct population of thrombotic microangiopathy patients. Transfusion 2004;44:146-150.

184. Jin M, Casper TC, Cataland SR et al. Relationship between ADAMTS13 activity in clinical remission and the risk of TTP relapse. Br.J.Haematol. 2008;141:651-658.

185. Peyvandi F, Lavoretano S, Palla R et al. ADAMTS13 and anti-ADAMTS13 antibodies as markers for recurrence of acquired thrombotic thrombocytopenic purpura during remission. Haematologica 2008;93:232-239.

186. Hovinga JA, Vesely SK, Terrell DR, Lammle B, George JN. Survival and relapse in patients with thrombotic thrombocytopenic purpura. Blood 2010;115:1500-1511.

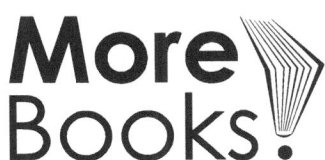

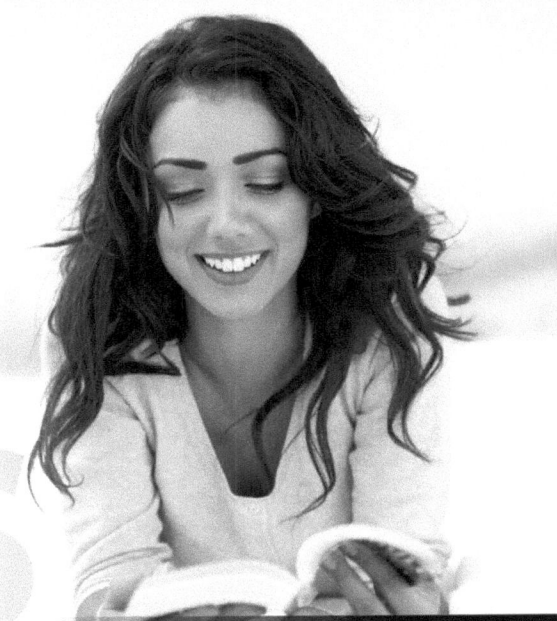

# i want morebooks!

Buy your books fast and straightforward online - at one of world's fastest growing online book stores! Environmentally sound due to Print-on-Demand technologies.

## Buy your books online at
## www.get-morebooks.com

Kaufen Sie Ihre Bücher schnell und unkompliziert online – auf einer der am schnellsten wachsenden Buchhandelsplattformen weltweit! Dank Print-On-Demand umwelt- und ressourcenschonend produziert.

## Bücher schneller online kaufen
## www.morebooks.de

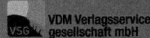 VDM Verlagsservicegesellschaft mbH
Heinrich-Böcking-Str. 6-8    Telefon: +49 681 3720 174    info@vdm-vsg.de
D - 66121 Saarbrücken        Telefax: +49 681 3720 1749   www.vdm-vsg.de

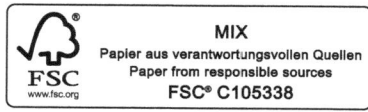

Printed by Books on Demand GmbH, Norderstedt / Germany